LONG-TERM HEMODIALYSIS

LONG-TERM HEMODIALYSIS

N.K. Man
Hôpital Necker, Département de Néphrologie, Paris, France

J. Zingraff
Hôpital Necker, Département de Néphrologie, Paris, France

and

P. Jungers
Hôpital Necker, Département de Néphrologie, Paris, France

Illustrated by Martine Netter

Kluwer Academic Publishers
Dordrecht / Boston / London

Library of Congress Cataloging-in-Publication Data
Man, N. K.
　　Long-term hemodialysis / by N.-K. Man, and J. Zingraff,
　and P. Jungers.
　　　　p.　　cm.
　　Includes index.
　　ISBN 0-7923-3477-9 (hb : alk. paper)
　　1. Hemodialysis.　2. Hemodialysis--Complications.　I. Zingraff,
Johanna.　II. Jungers, P.　III. Title.
　　[DNLM: 1. Hemodialysis.　2. Hemodialysis--adverse effects.
　3. Kidney Failure, Chronic--therapy.　4. Long-Term Care.　WJ 378
　M266L 1995]
　RC901.7.H45M355　1995
　617.4'61059--dc20
　DNLM/DLC
　for Library of Congress   95-14248
ISBN 0-7923-3477-9

Published by Kluwer Academic Publishers
P.O. Box 17, 3300 AA Dordrecht, The Netherlands.

Kluwer Academic Publishers incorporates
the publishing programmes of
D. Reidel, Martinus Nijhoff, Dr W. Junk and MTP Press.

Sold and distributed in the U.S.A. and Canada
by Kluwer Academic Publishers,
101 Philip Drive, Norwell MA 02061, U.S.A.

In all other countries, sold and distributed
by Kluwer Academic Publishers Group,
P.O. Box 322, 3300 AH Dordrecht, The Netherlands.

Printed on acid-free paper

All Rights Reserved
© 1995 Kluwer Academic Publishers

No part of the material protected by this copyright notice may be reproduced or utilized in any form or by any means, electronic or mechanical, including photocopying, recording, or by any information storage and retrieval system, without written permission from the copyright owners.

Printed in the Netherlands

TABLE OF CONTENTS

Preface   xi

1. Causes and consequences of end-stage renal failure   1
   Epidemiology of chronic renal failure   1
      Types of renal disease leading to ESRD   1
      Incidence of renal diseases leading to ESRD   2
      Changing pattern of epidemiology   2
   The uremic syndrome   4
      Accumulation of low-molecular weight waste products   5
      Accumulation of middle molecular weight toxins   6
      Loss of hydroelectrolytic regulation   7
      Loss of hormonal functions   7
   Indications for initiating dialysis therapy   7
      Criteria for initiation of dialysis   8
      Preparation of the patient for regular dialysis treatment   9

2. Basic principles of hemodialysis   11
   Transport mechanisms   11
      Diffusion (or conduction)   11
      Convection (or ultrafiltration)   12
      Adsorption   13
   Modalities of solute transport   13
      Solute transport in hemodialysis   14
      Solute transport in hemofiltration   14
      Solute transport in hemodiafiltration   15
   Evaluation of dialyzer performances   16
      Clearance   16

Dialysance	17
Ultrafiltration	18
Contribution of convection to the overall solute transport	19
Assessment of solute mass removal	20

3. Blood access — 22

Standard arteriovenous fistula	22
Alternative methods	23
Autogenous vein grafts	23
Other graft material	24
Occasional devices	24
Complications and long-term management of arteriovenous devices	25
Stenosis and clotting	25
Bacterial infections	26
Excessive flow rate	27
Temporary access methods	27

4. Dialysis equipment — 29

Dialyzers	29
Flat plate dialyzers	29
Hollow-fiber dialyzers	29
Large surface area dialyzers and high flux dialyzers	30
Residual blood volume	31
Dialyzer thrombogenicity	31
Reuse of dialyzers	31
Dialysis membranes	31
Chemical structure	31
Permeability characteristics	32
Dialysate delivery system	33
Dialysate preparation	33
Monitoring	35
Hemodiafiltration monitor	35
Computerized monitoring	35
Disinfection of dialysate delivery system	36
Dialysate composition	36
Water treatment	39

5. Biocompatibility — 42

Activation of blood components	42
Complement activation	42
Clinical consequences of complement activation	44

	Activation of blood coagulation	45
	Acute anaphylactoid reactions	45
	Long-term consequences of bioincompatibility	47

6. Adequacy of hemodialyis, nutrition, and dialysis prescription — 49
- Quantification of dialysis efficacy — 49
  - Urea kinetic modeling: the Kt/V concept — 49
  - Correlations between Kt/V (urea) and outcome — 51
- Nutritional parameters of dialysis adequacy — 52
  - Assessment of nutritional status: the PCR concept — 52
  - Correlations between nutritional parameters and outcome — 53
  - Interrelationship between URR and PCR — 53
- Choice of adequate dialysis duration — 54
  - Kt/V-based calculation of dialysis duration — 54
  - Adequate dialysis prescription — 56
- Dietary prescription to the hemodialysis patient — 57
  - Calorie-protein requirements — 57
  - Sodium and water intake — 58
  - Nutritional prescription — 58
- Integrated dialysis prescription — 59

7. Management of the dialysis patient — 61
- First hemodialysis session — 61
- Monitoring of later sessions — 62
  - Vascular connexion — 62
  - Heparinization — 62
  - Fluid removal by ultrafiltration — 63
  - Patient's activity and meals during hemodialysis — 63
  - End of dialysis and blood restitution — 64
  - Clinical surveillance of the dialysis session — 64
- Technical hazards during hemodialysis sessions — 64
  - Hemodialysis-related hypotension — 65
  - Other intradialytic complications — 66
- Interdialytic complications — 67
- Modalities of hemodialysis treatment — 67
- Long-term surveillance of the dialysis patient — 68

8. Cardiovascular and neurological problems — 69
- Hypertension — 70
- Cardiac dysfunction in uremia — 71
  - Mechanisms of cardiac dysfunction — 71
  - Clinical consequences and management — 72

Atherosclerosis and coronaropathy	73
Factors of accelerated atherosclerosis	73
Clinical expression and diagnostic procedures	73
Therapeutic management	74
Pericarditis	74
Valvular heart disease	75
Uremic neurological involvement	76
Uremic encephalopathy	76
Uremic polyneuropathy	76
Iatrogenic manifestations	76
Aluminum encephalopathy	77
Cerebrovascular accidents	77
9. Immunologic and hematologic disorders	**78**
Immune system dysregulation	78
Immunodeficiency	79
Immunoactivation	79
Bacterial infections	81
Staphylococcal infections	81
Gram-negative organisms	81
Unusual infections	82
Viral hepatitis	82
Hepatitis B	83
Hepatitis C	83
Anemia and erythropoetin therapy	84
Mechanisms and consequences of anemia	84
Treatment of anemia	85
Management of EPO therapy	86
Hemostasis disorders	87
Platelet dysfunction in uremics	87
Bleeding tendency	87
10. Bone and joint problems	**88**
Secondary hyperparathyroidism	89
Pathogenesis	89
Clinical presentation	90
Prophylactic treatment	91
Treatment of overt secondary hyperparathyroidism	92
Aluminum-related osteomalacia	93
Pathophysiology and diagnosis	93
Treatment of Aluminum accumulation	94
Adynamic bone disease	94

    Beta 2-microglobulin amyloidosis   94
        Clinical manifestations   95
        Pathogenesis and risk factors   95
    Other osteoarticular problems   96
        Soft tissue calcifications   96
        Secondary gout   97
        Osteoporosis and bone fluorosis   97
        Destructive spondylarthropathy   98

11. Other clinical problems   99
    Endocrine disorders   99
    Metabolic disorders   100
    Dermatological problems   100
        Uremic pruritus   100
        Bullous dermatoses   101
    Gastrointestinal complications   102
        Functional disorders   102
        GI bleeding   102
        Other digestive complications   103
    Complications in the diseased kidneys   103
        Acquired cystic kidney disease   103
        Kidney stones   104
    Psychological problems   104
    Dialysis in children   104
        Technical problems   105
        Metabolic problems   105
    Dialysis in the elderly   106
    Dialysis in the diabetic patient   106
        Growing incidence of diabetic ESRF   106
        Management of the diabetic dialysis patient   107

12. Outcome and economics   108
    Results of maintenance hemodialysis   108
        Survival of patients on hemodialysis   108
        Quality of life and rehabilitation   109
    Economics of dialysis therapy   110
        Increasing needs of dialysis therapy   110
        The cost of dialysis therapy   111

Literature for further reading   113

Subject index   121

PREFACE

Major advances in both the technology and the medical knowledge of maintenance hemodialysis have been made since the early stages of such treatment in the 60s. Hemodialysis is now an established therapeutic method, and the time has come to present an up-to-date approach to all its technical and medical aspects.

We adopted a simple and concise style with a clear design and a large number of tables and illustrations, so that not only health professionals but patients themselves can easily understand the essentials of hemodialysis.

In addition to the most recent technical developments of hemodialysis, particular attention is given to biocompatibility, adequacy of dialysis and patient nutrition. The many clinical problems encountered in the dialysis patient have been especially emphasized, since proper management may prevent most uremia-related complications. Indeed, chronic hemodialysis consists not only of providing the patient with safe and well-tolerated dialysis sessions but also of maintaining good general condition, adequate nutritional status and well-being in the long term.

All of us have worked in the field of nephrology and hemodialysis at Necker Hospital for more than 25 years, and several of our very first patients are still enjoying life thanks to hemodialysis. We hope that our experience will be of help to nephrologists, renal nurses and technicians in training so that they can offer their patients, through optimal dialysis, long survival with the best possible quality of life and rehabilitation.

N.K. Man, MD
J. Zingraff, MD
P. Jungers, MD

CAUSES AND CONSEQUENCES OF END-STAGE RENAL FAILURE

The term "uremia" encompasses the sum of clinical and biochemichal disorders resulting from a severe reduction in kidney functions. Blood chemistry alterations develop early in the course of chronic renal failure and progressively increase in parallel to the reduction in active nephron mass. By contrast, overt clinical manifestations of uremic toxicity develop much later, at the very advanced stage of renal failure, usually when glomerular filtration rate (GFR) falls below 10 ml/min, i.e., ten times lower than normal.

> Beyond that point, defined as end-stage renal disease (ESRD), preservation of homeostasis is no longer possible and supportive treatment by dialysis or transplantation is needed to maintain life by replacing the excretory and regulatory functions of the diseased kidneys.

Epidemiology of chronic renal failure

Types of renal disease leading to ESRD

> Even if the same types of renal disease are encountered in every part of the world, their respective incidence varies widely among the various countries.

The main types of renal disease leading to ESRD are glomerular diseases (the most frequent now being IgA nephropathy, especially in Eastern countries), diabetic nephropathy (presently the most prevalent in the

United States), hypertensive nephrosclerosis, polycystic kidney disease, chronic interstitial nephritis, reflux nephropathy, obstructive nephropathy, and renal involvement as part of systemic diseases (such as systemic lupus erythematosus, vasculitis, and multiple myeloma).

> Most renal diseases progress slowly to ESRD and allow optimal preparation of the patient for supportive therapy. Some, however, have a very rapid course or are lately diagnosed, and therefore do not allow such preparation.

> Although the specific cause of chronic renail failure has little influence on the indication and management of maintenance dialysis, it is important to consider in the perspective of kidney transplantation

Incidence of renal diseases leading to ESRD

The present distribution of the various renal diseases identified as causes of ESRD in the USA, Japan and Europe is shown on Figure 1–1.

Diabetic nephropathy and hypertensive nephrosclerosis are preponderant in United States, whereas chronic glomerulonephritis is the leading cause in Japan. A more balanced pattern is observed in European countries with chronic glomerulonephritis accounting for 25%, hypertensive nephrosclerosis for 14%, and diabetic nephropathy for about 14%. Such disparities reflect differences in the incidence of acquired renal diseases, especially glomerular diseases, and in the prevalence of diabetes and essential hypertension among the various countries.

> In parallel, the number of new patients reaching end-stage renal failure markedly varies among countries. Based on the most recent reports for the years 1991–1994, the annual incidence of ESRD in the general population is clearly higher in the USA ($\approx$ 180/million population) and in Japan ($\approx$ 150/million) than in Europe ($\approx$ 80/million) (Figure 1–2).

Changing pattern of epidemiology

In the early days of maintenance hemodialysis, this therapy was restricted to young adults without severe extrarenal complications, who were expected to have the most potential for achieving full rehabilitation. Today, in most industrialized countries, enough facilities exist so that no selection is made based on type of renal disease, age, sex, economic status or comorbid conditions.

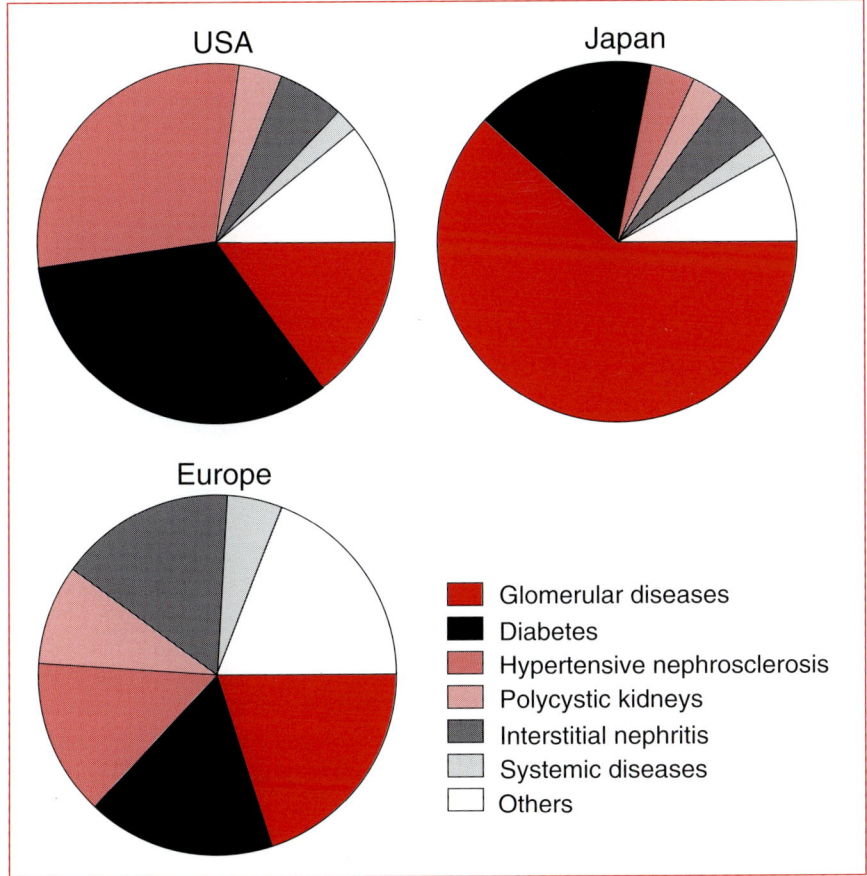

Figure 1-1: Distribution of renal diseases leading to ESRD in Europe, Japan and the USA.

> Accordingly, there has been a relentless increase in the mean age of patients accepted for dialysis.

Whereas the proportion of patients aged 65 years or more at start of dialysis, according to the European Dialysis and Transplant Association annual reports, was 9% in 1977 and 17% in 1982, it rose to 25% in 1987 and reached 38% in 1992 (Figure 1–3). The same trend, even more marked, is observed in the USA.

> The proportion of new patients with diabetic nephropathy is also constantly increasing in the USA (especially in Blacks) and in Northern European countries.

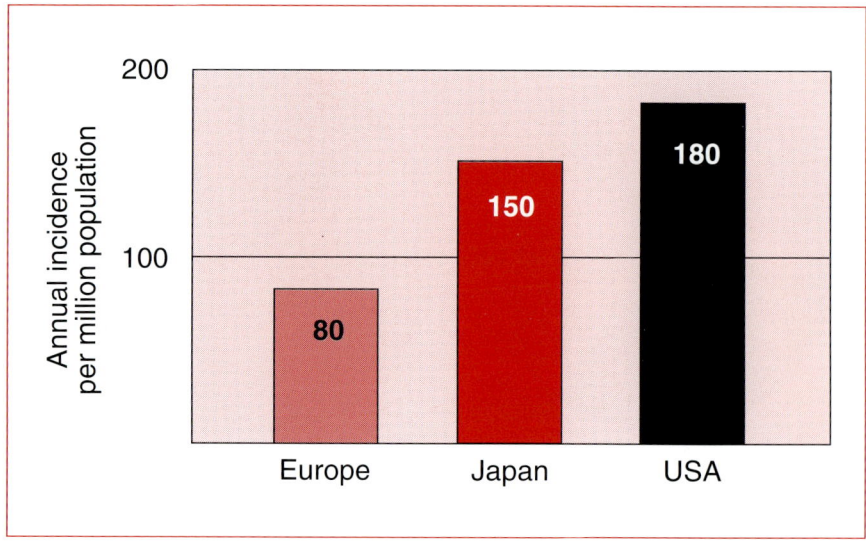

Figure 1-2: Annual incidence of ESRD in Europe, Japan and the USA.

As a result, a number of patients presently accepted on dialysis programs add the adverse effects of age and multiorgan involvement to the consequences of uremia itself, leading to greater morbidity and mortality, as well as more difficult management.

The uremic syndrome

Clear knowledge of the consequences of the loss of renal functions is needed to understand how maintenance hemodialysis acts and what are its possibilities and limitations.

Normal kidneys assume three main functions: excretion of waste products of nitrogen metabolism, regulation of water and electrolyte balance, and specific endocrine functions.

Because maintenance hemodialysis is a purely physical process, it can substitute for the first two functions, but endocrine, metabolic and immunologic disturbances that accompany loss of renal function cannot be corrected by dialysis, but require specific pharmacologic treatment.

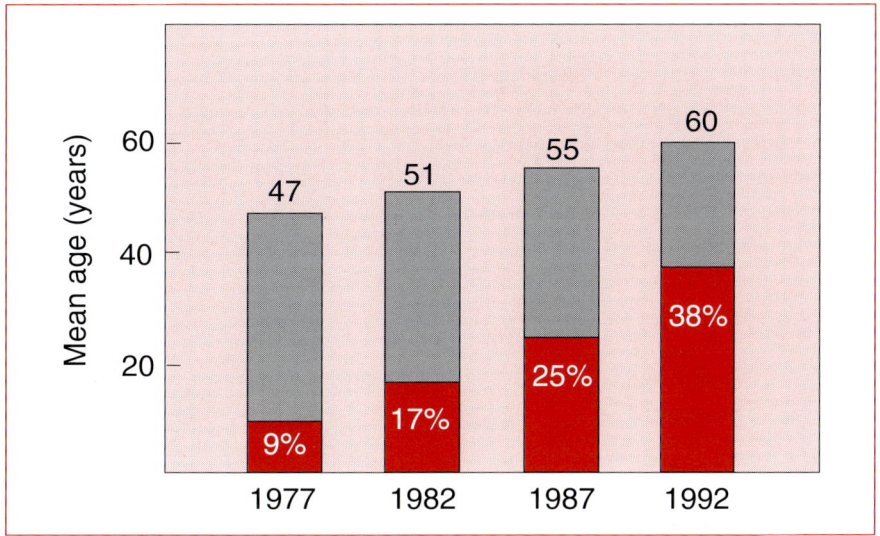

Figure 1-3: Relentless increase in the mean age of patients, and in the proportion of patients aged >65 years at start of dialysis therapy in Europe from 1977 to 1992 (EDTA-ERA annual reports).

Accumulation of low-molecular weight waste products

The kidneys are the main route for eliminating urea and other nitrogenous compounds resulting from protein catabolism. At comparable protein intake, the uremic patient produces and excretes daily the same amount of urea as does a subject with normal renal function, but at the price of an increased concentration in plasma. Such accumulation is proportional to functional nephron loss and reflects the degree of renal impairment.

Urea is quantitatively the most abundant of nitrogen (N) waste products. Its generation depends on protein intake. The catabolism of 6.25 g of protein leads to 2 g of urea, containing 1 g of N. As long as blood urea concentration is under 40 mmol/l, or blood urea nitrogen (BUN) less than 120 mg/dl, no clinical toxicity ensues. Higher concentrations are associated with anorexia, nausea, vomiting and drowsiness.

Creatinine and uric acid accumulate in plasma in inverse proportion to GFR. They exert no direct toxicity, but accumulation of uric acid may provoke gouty attacks.

Of note, maintenance hemodialysis restores to the patient an averaged urea clearance of about 15 ml/min/1.73m^2

Accumulation of middle molecular weight toxins

A number of components with a molecular weight (MW) ranging between 300 and 12000 daltons ("middle-molecular weight" toxins) also accumulate in uremics. Due to lower diffusibility, their elimination across dialysis membranes is much slower than for low MW solutes. Some are hormones or peptides, other are various organic compounds. More than 80 molecules have been incriminated as uremic toxins. The most important in view of possible deleterious effects are indicated in Table 1–1.

TABLE 1-1. Main molecules involved in uremic toxicity

	MW (d)	Deleterious effects
Low MW molecules		
Myoinositol	180	neurotoxicity
Purines (xanthines)	152	↓ calcitriol synthesis, anorexia
Oxalate	126	tissue deposition of calcium
Dimethylarginine	202	↓ nitric oxide synthesis
Middle MW molecules		
Peptides	variable	impaired monocyte function
Parathormone	9,424	↑ intracellular calcium
β-2 microglobulin	11,818	β2-mamyloidosis
Small molecules with "middle molecule" behaviour		
Methylguanidine	73	anorexia, vomiting
Guanidinosuccinic acid	175	↓ platelet aggregability
Indoxyl sulfate	251	↓ drug protein binding
Hippuric acid	179	↓ drug protein binding
Polyamines (spermine)	202	↓ erythropoiesis
Phenols and indoles	94	↓ activity of PMN and platelets
Carboxymethylpropyl-furanpropionic acid (CMPF)	240	↓ drug protein binding
Chloramines	variable	hemolysis
Homocysteine	135	atherogenesis

Adpated from Vanholder et al., Semin Nephrol 1994; 14: 205–218, with permission

> Uremic toxicity is multifactorial and no single uremic clinical manifestation can be attributed to a specific molecule.

Of note, some low MW molecules (such as guanidines or indoles), due to high protein binding, lipophilicity and/or multicompartmental distribution, may behave like larger molecules, therefore also requiring a longer dialysis time in order to be cleared.

> All toxins, whatever their MW, have to be adequately removed by hemodialysis. It results that the duration of dialysis sessions must be sufficient to allow diffusion of all molecules between body compartments and ensure adequate dialysis efficacy.

Loss of hydroelectrolytic regulation

Up to the very end stage of renal disease the kidneys remain able to maintain the electrolyte and water balance of the body through enhanced individual excretion of water and electrolytes by residual nephrons. However, when the number of functioning nephrons falls below 5 percent of normal, adaptation is no longer possible and only replacement therapy can maintain life.

After the start of maintenance hemodialysis, diuresis usually decreases, due to the reduction of the osmotic load of urea by dialysis. Urinary output usually falls below 500 ml per day and with time is often reduced to nil.

> In ESRD patients, water and electrolyte balance becomes almost entirely dependent on hemodialysis. Therefore, interdialytic intake of sodium, potassium and water should be reasonably limited in order to avoid excessive accumulation and the need for too rapid extraction during dialysis sessions.

Loss of hormonal functions

Normal kidneys produce erythropoietin, which stimulates erythrocyte production, and 1-α hydroxylase required to form calcitriol (1,25(OH)2 D3), the active form of vitamin D3. Their production is defective in ESRD patients. By contrast, enhanced activity of the renin-angiotensin axis often occurs, with specific deleterious consequences.

Indications for initiating dialysis therapy

The beginning of dialysis therapy should not be too delayed, in order to avoid symptoms of uremic toxicity and malnutrition, and not too advanced, when renal function is still sufficient. Because clinical symptoms of uremia do not closely parallel biochemical disorders, decision to start dialysis may be based on both clinical and biochemical parameters.

Criteria for initiation of dialysis

The ideal (and fortunately the most frequent) case is that of a patient with slowly progressive renal disease and regular nephrologic care. In this situation, uremic symptoms are often lacking throughout the follow-up.

> The decision to start dialysis will be based mainly on laboratory parameters. A generally accepted criterion is a GFR value comprised between 5 and 8 ml/min/1.73 m².

Creatinine clearance (Ccr) estimated from serum creatinine concentration, according to the Cockcroft and Gault formula, has been shown to closely parallel inulin clearance in patients with chronic renal failure and may be used as a simple simple means to estimate GFR for clinical purpose. The median of estimated Ccr at the time of dialysis initiation was 7 ml/min/1.73 m² in our current practice.

Finally, decision to start dialysis in asymptomatic patients will be taken when minor, but indisputable, symptoms of uremic toxicity arise, such as persistent nausea, vomiting, dyspnea, or unusually marked asthenia (Table 1–2).

TABLE 1-2. Indications for initiation of dialysis

Absolute indications
    Pericarditis
    Uremic encephalopathy or neuropathy
    Pulmonary edema and fluid overload unresponsive to usual measures
    Refractory hypertension
    Persistent vomiting
    Blood urea above 40 mmol/l (BUN > 120 mg/dl)
    Serum creatinine above 900 µmol/l (> 10 mg/dl)

Elective indications
    GFR (or estimated creatinine clearance*) between 5 and 8 ml/min/1.73m²
    Recent onset of nausea, anorexia, vomiting and/or marked asthenia
    Protein intake spontaneously falling under 0.7 g/kg/day

* according to the Cockcroft and Gault formula [Nephron 1976; 16: 31–41]

> High levels of urea or creatinine and/or severe clinical manifestations, especially uncontrolled hypertension, fluid overload or pericarditis, are absolute indications to start dialysis immediately.

Preparation of the patient for regular dialysis treatment

> Psychological preparation of the patient is fundamental. Long before the predictable initiation of dialysis, the patient should be informed of the future need for regular dialysis treatment.

The basic concept should be explained, particularly the indefinite duration of treatment unless transplantation is performed, but also the expected improvement in physical status and activity. Psychological support should be provided to overcome the inevitable psychological trauma of facing the constraint of indefinite treatment.

Technical aspects of patient's preparation involve timely creation of vascular access, preferably several months before the anticipated beginning of dialysis, in order to allow sufficient maturation of the arteriovenous fistula.

> It is recommended that a fistula should be created as soon as serum creatinine level reaches 600 µmol/l (about 7 mg/dl), and even sooner in female, aged or diabetic patients, and in patients with a poor venous network.

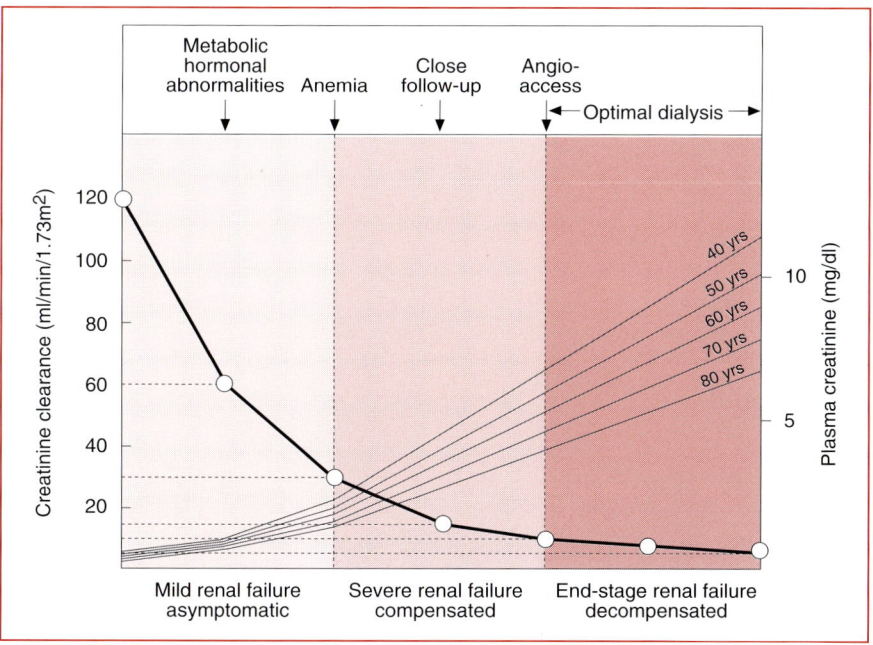

Figure 1-4: Progression of chronic renal failure and criteria for initiating maintenance hemodialysis.

Another important precaution is to start vaccination against hepatitis B virus before initiation of dialysis. The steps of patients' preparation are schematically represented on Figure 1–4.

Possibilities of renal transplantation should be evaluated in every patient especially in subjects under 65–70 years of age.

> Initiating dialysis before uremic complications and malnutrition occur is the best means of avoiding short-term mortality and morbidity and achieving rapid improvement in the quality of life, and socio-professional rehabilitation of uremic patients.

BASIC PRINCIPLES OF HEMODIALYSIS

Hemodialysis is a treatment which aims to remove accumulated metabolic waste products and to correct blood electrolyte composition by means of an exchange between patient's blood and a dialysate fluid mimicking normal extracellular fluid, across a semi-permeable membrane (Figure 2–1).

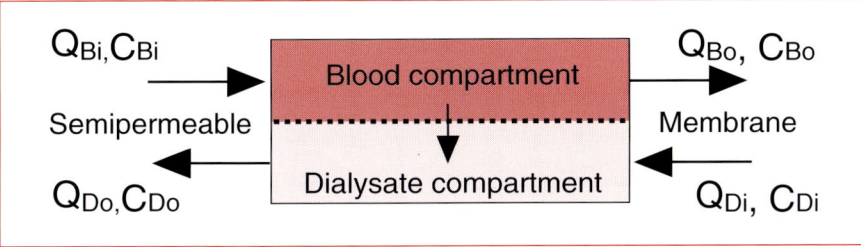

Figure 2-1: Schematic representation of an hemodialyzer. Note the counter-current circulation of blood and dialysate on each side of the semi-permeable membrane.

Transport mechanisms

Transport of solutes and water involves two mechanisms, diffusion and convection.

Diffusion (or conduction)

Diffusion is defined as the spontaneous passive transport of solutes from blood to dialysate (and vice versa, i.e., backdiffusion) across the dialysis membrane (Figure 2–2). The rate of diffusive transport depends upon the dif-

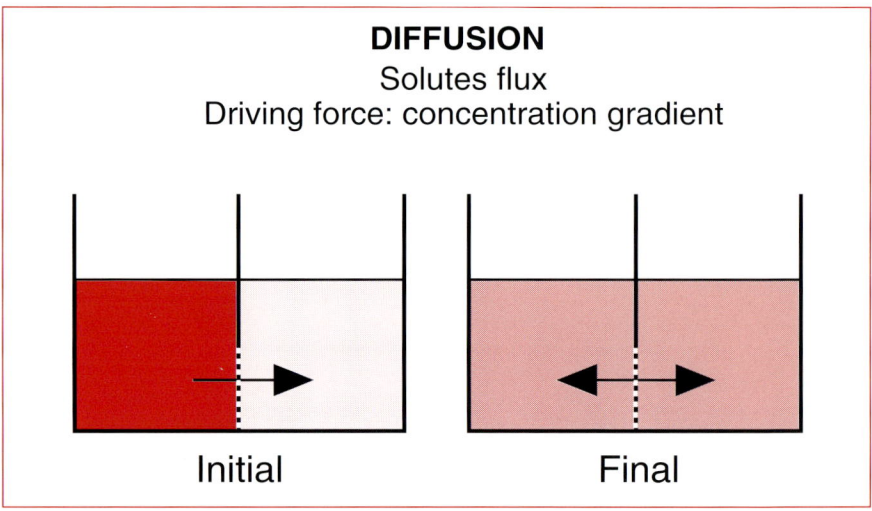

Figure 2-2: Schematic representation of the diffusive mechanism of solute transport.

fusion coefficients of the solute in blood, in membrane and in dialysate, the surface area of the membrane and the concentration difference across the membrane.

Thus, conductive mass transfer per unit membrane area is the result of the driving force (concentration difference) relative to the resistance to transfer (R_T), which is the sum of blood side resistance (R_B), membrane resistance (R_M) and dialysate side resistance (R_D).

$$R_T = R_B + R_M + R_D$$

> The velocity of a molecule in solution is inversely proportional to its molecular weight (MW). Consequently, the transport rate of low MW solutes is higher than that of high MW solutes.

Convection (or ultrafiltration)

Convection is the simultaneous transport of solvent and solutes from the blood compartment to the dialysate compartment (and vice versa, i.e., backfiltration) across the dialysis membrane (Figure 2–3). The rate of convective transport depends upon the hydraulic permeability, the sieving coefficient of the solute and the surface area of the membrane, the solute concentration in blood and the pressure gradient across the membrane.

The hydraulic permeability coefficient and the sieving coefficients are characteristics specific to a given membrane and depend upon the diameter

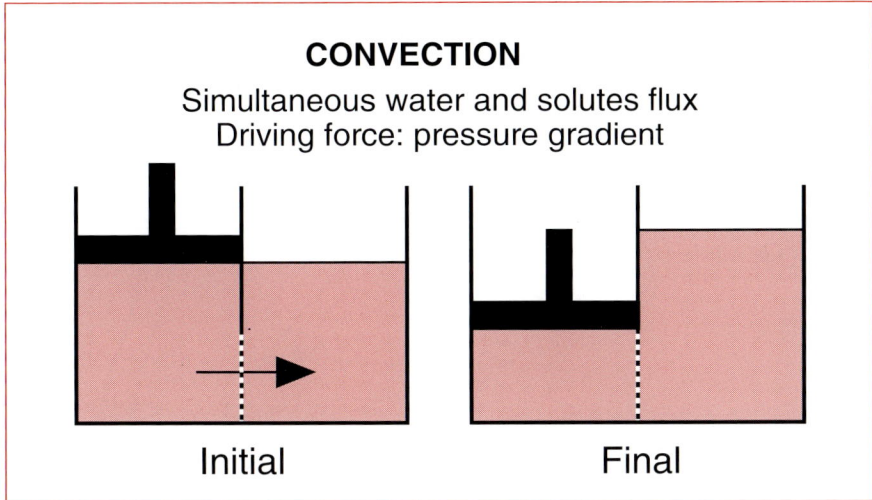

Figure 2-3: Schematic representation of the convective mechanism of water and solute transport.

of membrane pores and the number of pores per unit membrane area. High-permeability membranes now have sieving coefficients close to natural kidney glomerular barrier (Figure 2–4). The sieving coefficient for any solute is the ratio of its concentration in the filtrate to that in the plasma water.

> The effective transmembrane pressure is the difference between hydrostatic pressure and osmotic pressure. The latter is mostly determined by the oncotic pressure (about 30 mmHg) of blood proteins which cannot pass through the dialysis membrane.

Adsorption

To some extent, proteins such as albumin, fibrin, β2-microglobulin, fragments of activated human complement and cytokines such as IL-1 and TNFα are adsorbed onto the dialysis membrane. This contributes partly to their removal from blood. Protein adsorption depends upon the hydrophobic nature of the membrane.

Modalities of solute transport

The relative role of diffusion and convection in solute transport differs whether solute removal is achieved by hemodialysis, hemofiltration or hemodiafiltration.

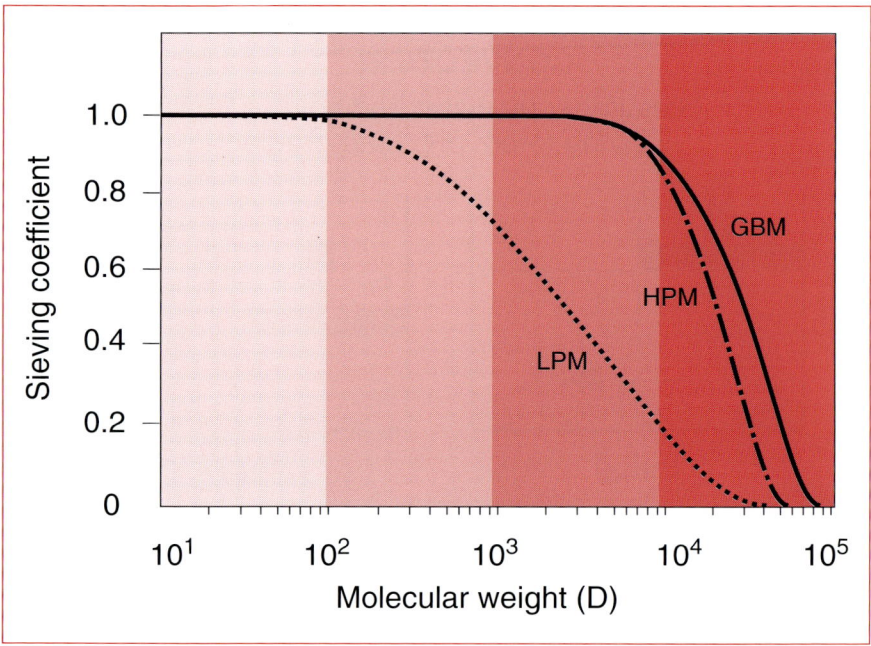

Figure 2-4: Compared sieving coefficients of low-permeability (LPM) and high-permeability (HPM) membranes, and of the natural glomerular barrier (GBM).

Solute transport in hemodialysis (figure 2–5a)

Transport of most solutes is diffusive whereas transport of sodium and fluid is mostly convective. Ultrafiltration flow rate is the main mechanism by which both water and sodium accumulated between dialysis sessions are removed from the body.

Solute transport in hemofiltration (figure 2–5b)

Transport of solutes is purely convective. The rate of solute removal is equal to the filtration rate times the solute concentration in the filtrate. Solute concentration in the filtrate is equal to the solute concentration in the plasma times the sieving coefficient.

At low transmembrane pressures, the filtration rate increases linearly with pressure gradient. At higher pressures, the filtration rate reaches a plateau where cells and proteins are concentrated at the surface of the membrane and limit the flux. To increase further the filtration rate, the blood flow rate should be increased (Figure 2–6).

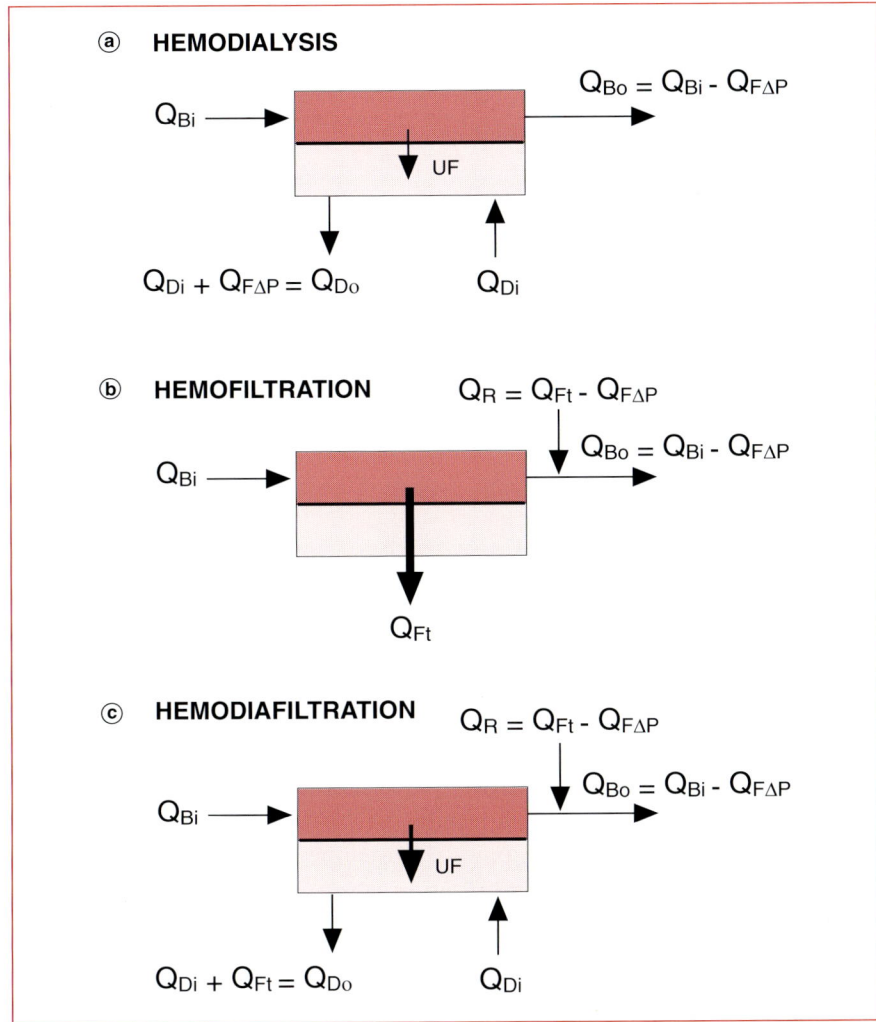

Fig. 2-5: Schematic representation of the mechanisms of solute transport by hemodialysis, hemofiltration and hemodiafiltration.

To prevent excessive removal of fluid, sterile and nonpyrogenic substitution fluid similar to dialysate composition is infused in the blood line at a flow rate of 10 to 15 L/hr, either upstream of the hemofilter (predilution mode) or usually downstream of the hemofilter (postdilution mode).

Solute transport in hemodiafiltration (figure 2–5c)

To combine the advantages of hemodialysis and hemofiltration, transport of solutes in hemodiafiltration is both diffusive for efficient removal of

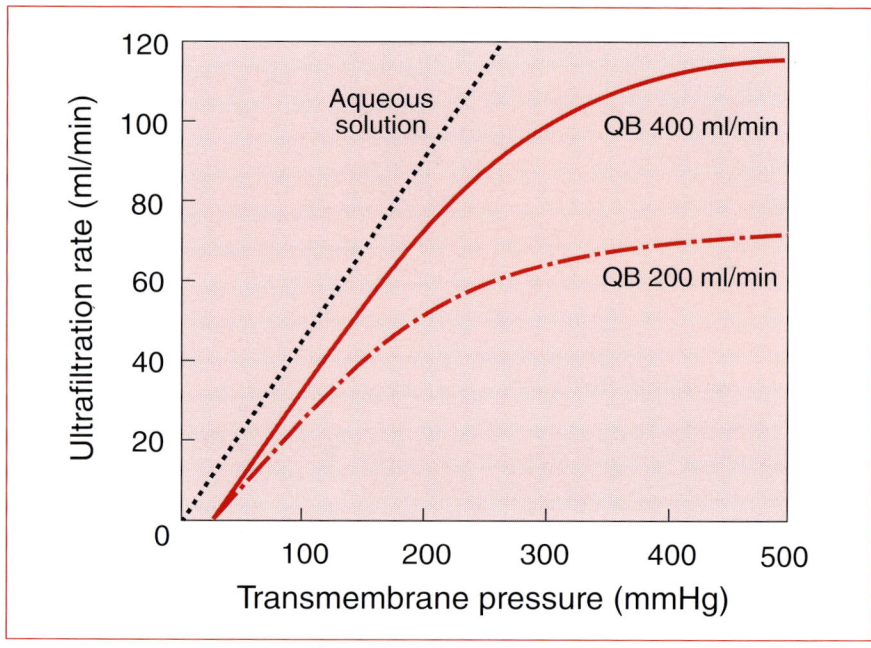

Figure 2-6: Interrelations between ultrafiltration rate and transmembrane pressure gradient, and the influence of blood flow rate.

small MW solutes, and convective for efficient removal of high MW solutes. The infusion flow rate is usually 5 to 10 L/hr.

Other methods which combine diffusive transport and convective transport include push-pull hemofiltration where periods of hemofiltration alternate with periods of backfiltration, paired-filtration dialysis where hemofiltration and hemodialysis operate in series, and biofiltration where base-free dialysate is used with sodium bicarbonate as substitution fluid.

Evaluation of dialyzer performances

Similar to the clearance concept from renal physiology, the overall solute transport by the artificial kidney may be expressed in terms of either clearance or dialysance.

Clearance

Clearance (C) is defined as the amount of solute (Js) removed from the blood per unit of time divided by the incoming blood concentration (CBi) and represents the volumetric rate at which blood is cleared of solute.

$$C = \frac{J_S}{C_{Bi}}$$

Dialysance

Dialysance (D) is defined as the amount of solute removed from the blood per unit of time (Js) divided by the concentration difference between incoming blood and incoming dialysate (CBi − CDi).

$$D = \frac{J_S}{C_{Bi} - C_{Di}}$$

Clearance and dialysance can be defined in terms of the inlet and outlet blood (Q_{Bi} and Q_{Bo}) and dialysate (Q_{Di} and Q_{Do}) flow rates, and the inlet and outlet blood (C_{Bi} and C_{Bo}) and dialysate (C_{Di} and C_{Do}) solute concentrations. The solute mass balance across the dialyzer in steady state can be written as follows:

$$(Q_{Bi} \times C_{Bi}) - (Q_{Bo} \times C_{Bo}) = (Q_{Di} \times C_{Di}) - (Q_{Do} \times C_{Do})$$

Thus clearance can be expressed as

$$C = \frac{(Q_{Bi} \times C_{Bi}) - (Q_{BO} \times C_{BO})}{C_{Bi}}$$

and dialysance as

$$D = \frac{(Q_{Bi} \times C_{Bi}) - (Q_{Bo} \times C_{Bo})}{C_{Bi} - C_{Di}}$$

For the case of single pass dialysate, and $C_{Di} = 0$, clearance is equal to dialysance. If the ultrafiltration rate is low, Q_{Bo} and Q_{Do} are not different from Q_{Bi} and Q_{Di}, and the equation for clearance can be simplified as follows:

$$C = \frac{C_{Bi} - C_{Bo}}{C_{Bi}} \times Q_B$$

> Clearance and dialysance are parameters that focus on the removal of solutes from the blood stream. Clearance is the most meaningful value since it characterizes the artificial kidney as part of the total body clearance, in analogy with the natural kidneys. Dialysance can be used for comparing overall solute removal capacities of a given dialyzer at specified blood and dialysate flow rates.

Solute clearance decreases with increasing solute molecular weight (Figure 2–7a). Clearance of low molecular weight solutes such as urea (MW 60 D) and creatinine (MW 113 D) increases with blood flow rate, whereas blood flow rate has little effect on high molecular weight solutes such as Vitamin B12 (MW 1355 D) (Figure 2–7b).

Ultrafiltration

The ultrafiltration rate (Q_F) is defined as the volumetric flow rate of solvent across the membrane per unit of time and is equal to the difference between the blood flow entering (Q_{Bi}) and leaving (Q_{Bo}) the dialyzer and, symmetrically, between the dialysate flow leaving (Q_{Do}) and entering (Q_{Di}) the dialyzer.

$$Q_F = Q_{Bi} - Q_{Bo} = Q_{Do} - Q_{Di}$$

The ultrafiltration rate depends upon the hydraulic permeability coefficient of the membrane (K_f), the effective membrane surface area (A) and the effective transmembrane pressure which is the difference between hydrostatic pressure (ΔP) and osmotic pressure ($\Delta \pi$):

$$Q_f = K_f \times A \times (\Delta P - \Delta \pi)$$

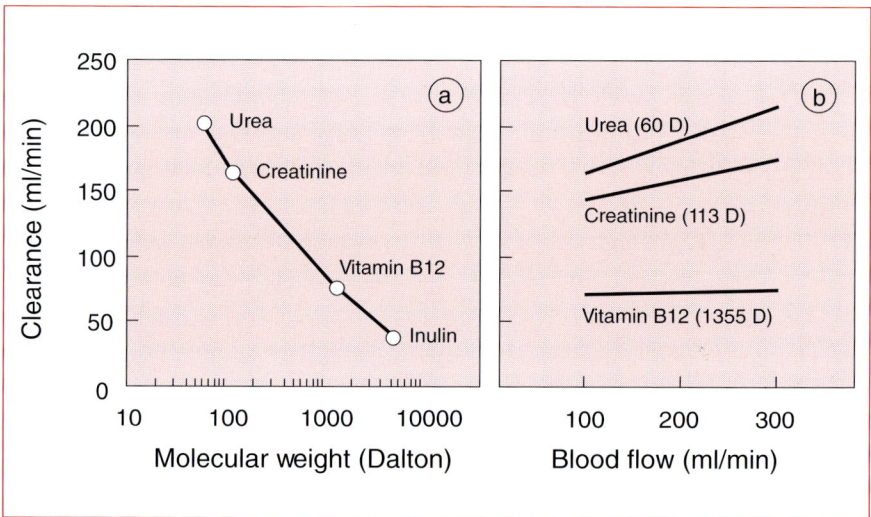

Figure 2-7: Solute clearance as a function of molecular weight (a) and of blood flow (b). Note the weak influence of blood flow on clearance of middle and high MW solutes.

BASIC PRINCIPLES OF HEMODIALYSIS

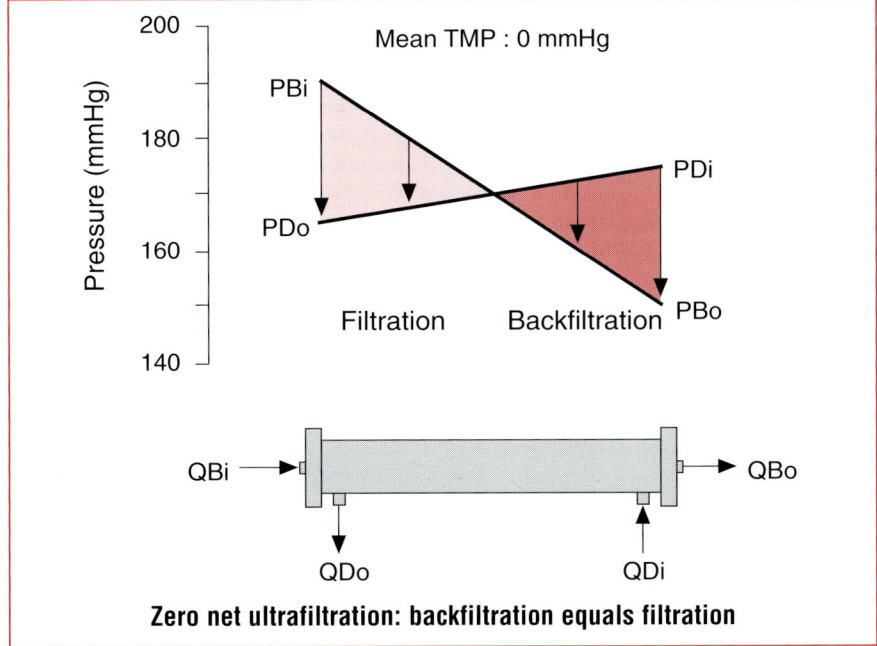

Figure 2-8: Mechanisms of filtration and backfiltration. Ultrafiltration occurs when PB>PD, whereas backfiltration takes place when PB<PD.

The mean hydrostatic pressure is equal to the algebraic sum of mean pressure in blood and dialysate compartments:

$$\Delta P = \frac{(P_{Bi} + P_{Bo})}{2} - \frac{(P_{Di} + P_{Do})}{2}$$

In order to avoid excessive fluid removal with high flux dialyzers, dialysate pressure must be maintained at a value which allows to yield the net ultrafiltration rate prescribed. This is usually achieved with a flow equalizer device. The net ultrafiltration rate is equal to the total ultrafiltration rate minus the backfiltration rate, as shown in Figure 2–8.

Contribution of convection to the overall solute transport

The contribution of convective transport to the overall solute transport is more prominent for high MW solutes than for low MW solutes.

To assess the relative contribution of convection to the overall solute transport, the sieving coefficients of the various solutes should be taken into account. For example, from the sieving coefficients and clearance data, with Q_B = 300 ml/min and Q_f= 10 ml/min, convective clearance C_C (Q_f × sieving coefficient) and the contribution of convection to the overall solute transport reflected by the C_C/C_{Total} ratio can be evaluated for low, middle or high MW solutes (Table 2–1).

Usually for an ultrafiltration flow rate of about 50 ml/min and for solutes with a sieving coefficient of about 1, when diffusion and convection cooperate for overall solute transport, total clearance (C_T) can be approximated as follows

$$C_T = C_D + Q_f \times \left(1 - \frac{C_D}{Q_B}\right)$$

where C_D is diffusive clearance for $Q_f = 0$.

TABLE 2-1. Relative contribution of convection to total solute clearance with respect to solute molecular weight

Solute (MW)	Urea (60D)	Vit.B12 (1355 D)	Inulin (5200 D)
Sieving coefficient	1.0	0.95	0.93
Total clearance (C_T), ml/min	205	77	40
Convective clearance (C_C), ml/min	10	9.5	9.3
C_C/C_T ratio	0.05	0.12	0.23

Assessment of solute mass removal

Mass transfer (N) of urea (or creatinine) during a dialysis session may be assessed in three ways.

1. Through whole blood clearance (K) determination according to the formula

    $$N = K \times C \times t_d$$

    where C is the logarithmic [($C_i - C_f$)/($LnC_i - LnC_f$)] or arithmetic [($C_i + C_f$)/2] mean of pre- (C_i) and postdialysis (C_f) blood concentration and t_d, dialysis duration.
2. By the difference between pre- (N_{pre}) and postdialysis (N_{post}) urea or creatinine mass, i.e.,

$$N = [C_i \times (TBW_f + V_{\Delta P})] - [C_f \times TBW_f]$$

where TBW_f is final total body water which is assumed to be equal to 58% of end-dialysis body weight and $V_{\Delta P}$, body weight loss.

Using these formulae, errors in the assessment of urea and creatinine mass removal could result from the underestimation of solute final concentration due to a rebound phenomenon, recirculation of blood in AV fistula, and from the possibly erroneous estimation of actual total body water.

3. By direct dialysate quantification. The latter is the most reliable method when effluent dialysate is totally collected in order to allow determination of the whole urea or creatinine mass extracted during a dialysis session. Mass transfer is equal to the solute concentration in dialysate times its volume. Total collection of dialysate, which is cumbersome and time consuming, may be replaced by aliquot collection.

Recently urea monitors have been designed which allow automated multiple dialysate sampling with on-line determination of urea concentration, thus providing direct quantification of the rate of urea removal during dialysis sessions.

3 BLOOD ACCESS

The long-term repeatability of hemodialysis sessions (usually 3 times per week) relies on a permanent vascular access allowing easy connection of patient's blood circuit to the dialyzer. Therefore a reliable, well tolerated blood access is obviously a prerequisite for successful maintenance hemodialysis.

Belding H. Scribner and coworkers conceived the first device of permanent blood access in the form of an external arteriovenous (AV) shunt. Subsequently the internal AV fistula proposed by Cimino and Brescia progressively substituted to the external device because of its better long-term patency.

Standard arteriovenous fistula

There is a now universal agreement that the method of choice for primary blood access is the subcutaneous arteriovenous (AV) radiocephalic fistula, connecting the radial artery to the cephalic vein at the wrist, preferentially in the non-dominant forearm.

> The most distal available site is to be used first in order to preserve maximal vessel length for future revision if needed.

Although the fistula initially described by Cimino and Brescia was a side-to-side anastomosis, surgeons today are more inclined to perform side-to-end (Figure 3–1) or eventually end-to-end anastomosis, to avoid swelling of the hand and excessive distension of the veins of the hand.

The optimal size of the anastomosis is matter of debate. Too small the

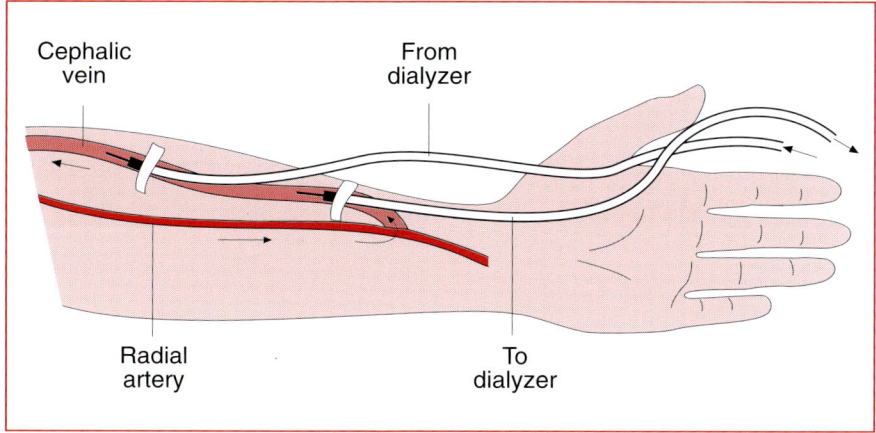

Figure 3-1: Standard arteriovenous (AV) fistula at the wrist.

risk of failure is high, too large the development may be complicated by an excessive blood flow rate ultimately leading to high-output cardiac failure. The anastomotic orifice should be nearly as large as the diameter of the nutrient artery. The optimal blood flow rate in the venous part of the fistula is around 700 ml/min.

Alternative methods

When repeated attempts to construct a radiocephalic AV fistula failed or when, from the very onset of dialysis therapy, no peripheral vessel access site is available, alternative techniques must be considered. A variety of so-called secondary access procedures can be proposed utilizing either human veins or prosthetic materials.

Autogenous vein grafts

The most widely used vein is the own saphenous vein of the patient, implanted in the arm in straight or in loop configuration (Figure 3–2a). The most distal possible artery should be chosen as nutrient vessel in order to limit the risk of excessive flow rate. The subcutaneous transposition of a previously arterialized deep vein of the arm or the thigh might be proposed as a variant of these techniques.

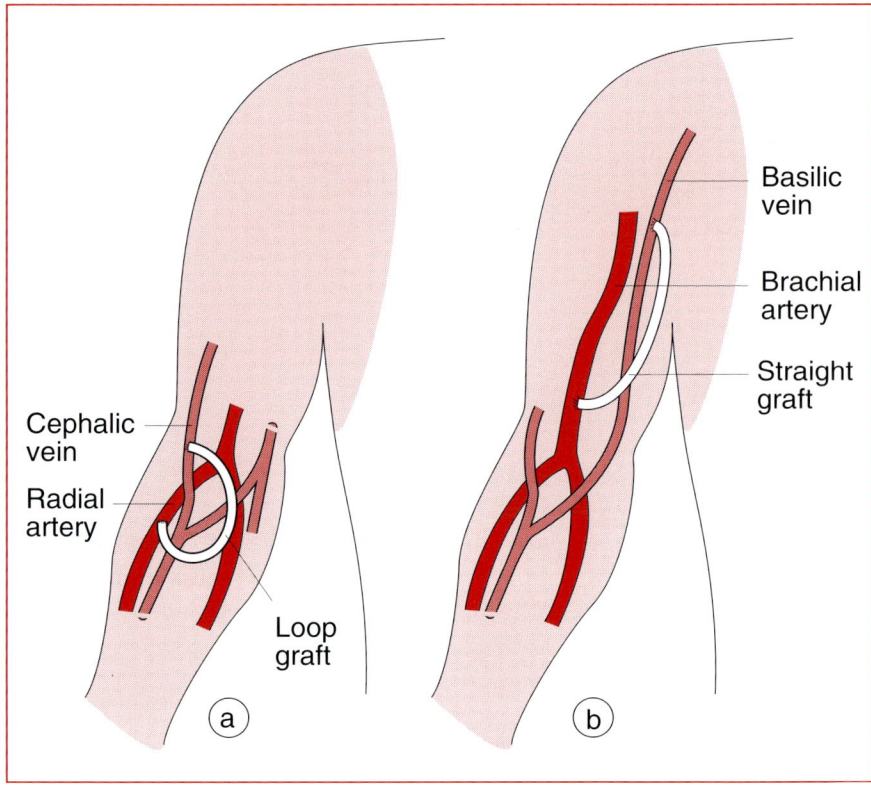

Figure 3-2: Loop configuration (a) or straight position (b) of an AV graft in the upper extremity.

Other graft material

Graft material other than autogenous veins includes allogenous veins (umbilical cord veins, or saphenous veins collected during stripping for varices), xenografts as the bovine carotid artery, or synthetic devices mainly composed of polytetrafluoroethylene (PTFE). All these graft materials may be used in the same configurations as are used autografts (Figure 3–2b).

Occasional devices

As an ultimate recourse, an arterial jump graft or a subcutaneously fixed humeral artery can be used as blood access, the latter especially when dilated by a previous homolateral AV fistula. Such a solution has no adverse effect on cardiac function, but the most frequent complication is the development of aneurysmal lesions.

The external Thomas shunt, placed between the femoral artery and the femoral vein has virtually been abandoned because of the incidence of dreadful complications potentially leading to leg amputation.

The Hemasite ® blood access device consists of a biocarbon implant mounted on a bovine graft or a PTFE vascular prosthesis. The self-sealing valve of the device allows blood access by disposable connectors and thus eliminates needle punctures. In spite of this advantage, this type of blood access exposes to the same complications as other prosthetic AV devices.

Complications and long-term management of arteriovenous devices

Stenosis and clotting

Clotting of the blood access, secondary to stenosis by intimal thickening, is the most frequent complication that may lead to fistula failure.It remains a major cause of morbidity and hospitalization cost in patients undergoing hemodialysis.

> Stenosis of the venous outflow will favour blood recirculation, decreasing the effectiveness of the dialysis.

Today, the fistula occlusion does not necessarily means loss of the access site. The patency can be reestablished by thrombolysis using fibrinolytic drugs and/or percutaneous transluminal angioplasty (PTA). Residual or recurrent stenoses can be redilated and eventually an endovascular stent can be placed (Figure 3–3). Such a stent does not preclude subsequent angioplasty when needed, even inside of the stent.

> Occlusion of the A-V fistula is generally a preventable event, provided that blood access is monitored vigilantly by regular surveillance of the venous return pressure during dialysis sessions and Doppler flow velocimetry assessment of the fistula.

When venous return pressure is increased, ultrasound detection of stenosis and eventually angiography should be performed. Early PTA may prevent repeated clotting of the fistula and may contribute to maintain long-term function of blood access.

> In spite of the most careful management, repeated clotting of the vascular access occurs in a small number of patients. Extensive

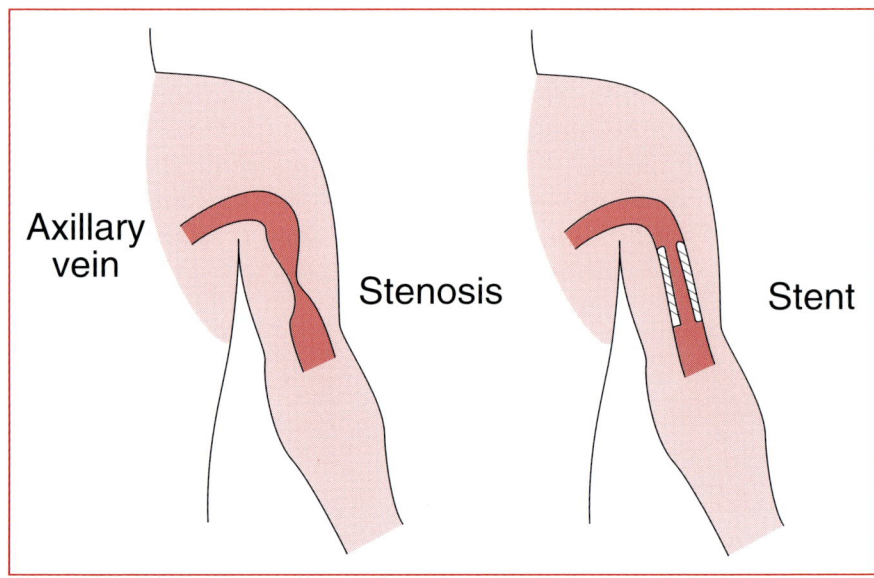

Figure 3-3: Angiographic aspect of venous stenosis of an AV fistula before and after percutaneous endoluminal angioplasty and stent implantation.

> coagulation studies should be performed in those subjects including determination of protein C, total and free protein S, search for circulating anticoagulant and for anticardiolipin antibodies. Permanent antivitamin K therapy may be indicated.

Bacterial infections

Bacterial infections occurring in hemodialysis patients are related to the vascular access in more than half of the cases. Infection rate is the highest for central catheters and the lowest for endogenous fistulae. The main consequence is the risk of developing septicemia and even endocarditis. The most commonly isolated micro-organisms in those patients are Staphylococcus aureus and Staphylococcus epidermidis. Septicemia may occur without evidence of local signs of infection. Treatment must associate local care to systemic antibiotics.

Percutaneous transluminal manipulation exposes to a high infectious risk and should therefore be performed under rigorously aseptic conditions as in surgery.

Excessive flow rate

> Excessive flow rate of the AV device may lead to high-output cardiac failure. Non-invasive flow measurements by ultrasonic Doppler velocimetry should be regularly performed together with cardiac echography, especially in patients who have a proximal AV access. A fistula with a flow rate over 1000 ml/min must be surgically reduced.

Complications of less frequent occurrence or of minor importance are listed in Table 3–1.

TABLE 3-1. Complications of vascular access

Stenosis of the anastomosis or the arterialized vein
Clotting (secondary or not to stenosis)
Infection (local or systemic)
Excessive blood flow (risk of high-output cardiac failure)
Distal ischemia (steal syndrome, favored by atherosclerosis)
Aneurysmal venous dilatation
Hemorrhage from ruptured aneurysm
Edema of the arm or leg, due to stenosis of a central vein
Local hematoma (post-puncture)
Infrequent: carpal tunnel syndrome
             arterial embolism
             small pulmonary emboli (symptomatic when infected)

Temporary access methods

> Central venous catheters are widely used in patients with end-stage renal failure in whom blood access has failed or was not created sufficiently in advance to be functioning when renal replacement therapy is required.

Two main routes are used: the femoral vein and the internal jugular vein. The femoral vein may be punctured repeatedly but usually no more than a few times. Permanent catheters are inserted inside of neck veins, preferentially fixed in a subcutaneous tunnel. The internal jugular vein should be preferred to the subclavian vein, since the incidence of post-catheter partial or total occlusion of the subclavian vein is unacceptably high, the internal jugular route being less traumatic. Silastic twin catheters allow adequate dialysis and are well tolerated (Figure 3–4). A double-lumen catheter also offers a satisfactory temporary access.

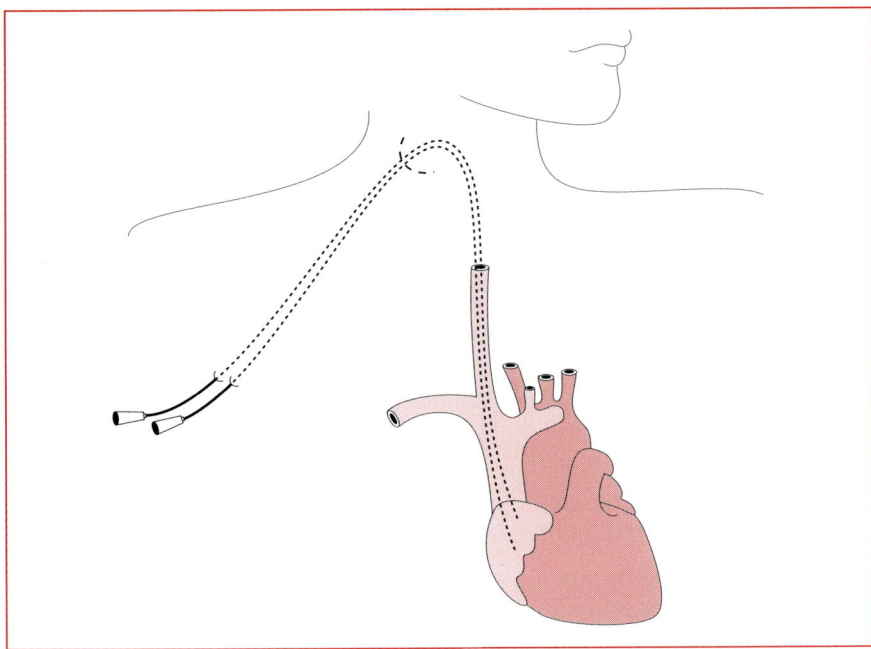

Figure 3-4: Schematic representation of twin catheters placed in the internal jugular vein via a subcutaneous tunnel.

> Tunnelized double-lumen or twin catheters in the jugular vein may be used for several weeks until an arteriovenous fistula is available, or even for months or years as permanent access in elderly or critically ill patients.

Whatever the success rate of these transitory solutions may be, a convenient, peripheral AV fistula created in time is the most comfortable solution for uremic patients who will be dependent for years and years on blood access.

4 DIALYSIS EQUIPMENT

Dialyzers

Only two types of dialyzers, flat plate and hollow fiber, are now currently in clinical use. They are supplied ready for use, sterilized by ethylene oxide, gamma rays or steam, and are intended to be fully disposable.

Flat plate dialyzers

Flat plate dialyzers are composed of a variable number of compartments in parallel separated by rigid support structures enclosing flat sheets of membrane (Figure 4–1). Blood flows between the membrane layers while dialysate flows counter-current across the support plates which have grooves or spaces for fluid flow. As blood and dialysate flow resistances are low, ultrafiltration is easily controlled and no or only minor backfiltration occurs.

Hollow-fiber dialyzers

Hollow-fiber dialyzers consist of 10–15,000 hollow fibers in a bundle, each end of which is embedded in a potting material. The fibers have an internal diameter of 200–300 µm and a wall thickness of 10–40 µm. The bundle is enclosed in a plastic jacket with ports for blood and dialysate lines. Blood flows within the fibers while dialysate flows counter-current on the outside of the fibers (Figure 4–1). Because of its high effective surface area to blood volume ratio and virtual lack of compliance, this design is theoretically the best. The dialyzer is also compact and easy to handle. All these advantages combine to make it the most popular dialyzer to date.

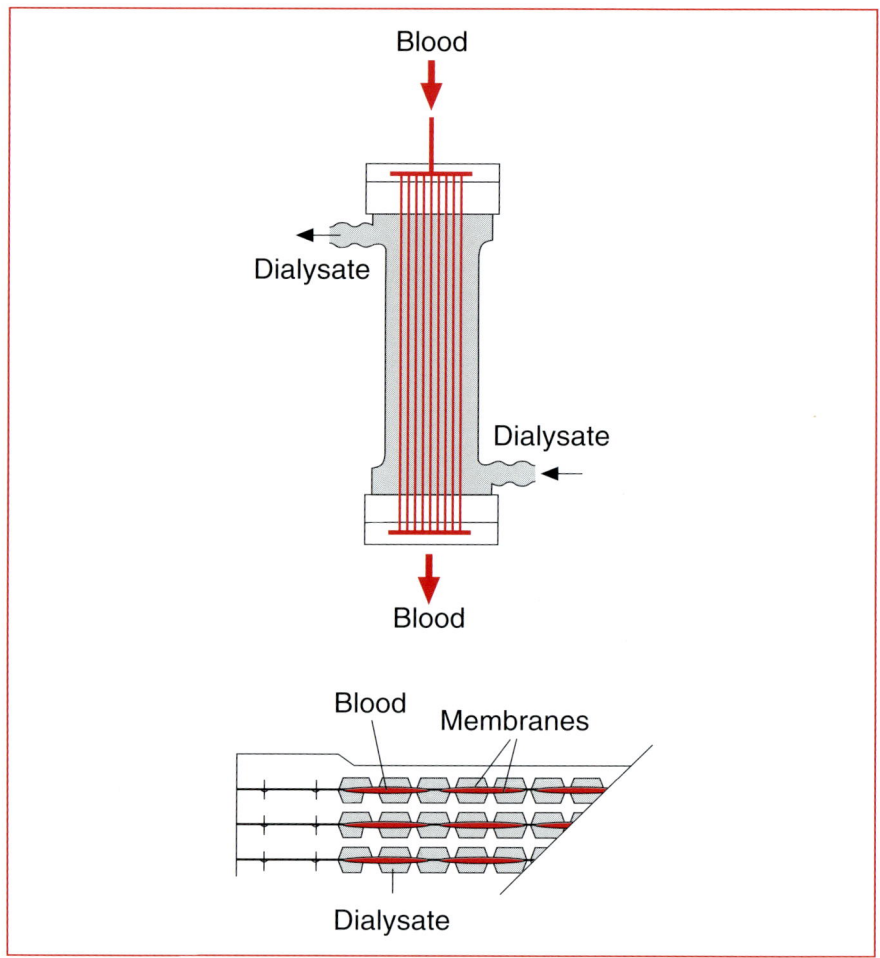

Figure 4-1: Schematic representation of hollow-fiber and flat-plate dialyzers.

Large surface area dialyzers and high flux dialyzers

Large surface area dialyzers (surface area up to 2 m^2) and high flux dialyzers (Kf up to 100 ml/hr/mmHg) were developed to increase solute mass removal and in order to reduce duration of dialysis sessions.

> Because of their high hydraulic permeability, the use of monitoring devices for the control of ultrafiltration flow rate is mandatory. Under such conditions, backfiltration occurs unless they are employed using hemofiltration or hemodiafiltration techniques.

Residual blood volume

> The residual blood volume depends upon the flow path geometry of the dialyzer, provided adequate heparinization is achieved, and upon the wash-back technique. Such blood loss is relatively small (about 1 ml) compared to other sources such as bleeding from fistulae sites and sampling for blood analysis.

Dialyzer thrombogenicity

Dialyzers and blood tubings are thrombogenic and require anti-coagulation, either of the patient or of the extracorporeal blood circuit. Inadequate heparinization may lead to significant thrombus formation which reduces the membrane surface area and consequently decreases the clearance and ultrafiltration characteristics of the dialyzers, and also results in blood loss for the patient.

A modified coagulation test, the whole blood activated partial thromboplastin time, is used to monitor heparin therapy during hemodialysis.

Reuse of dialyzers

Economic considerations have made the reuse of dialyzers desirable, particularly when using expensive devices such as large surface area or high flux dialyzers. Dialyzer reuse can be performed manually or automatically with reuse devices.

Adverse effects observed are specific to a given reuse procedure rather than inherent to reuse per se. Among the hazards is reinfusion into the patient of residual sterilant and/or blood products which have reacted with the chemicals used to clean and sterilize the dialyzer, thereby producing undesirable toxic and immunological reactions in the patient.

Dialysis membranes

Chemical structure

Dialysis membranes are designed to mimic permeability characteristics of the glomerular basement membrane. They are manufactured from a wide variety of polymers or copolymers. The membranes are extruded or cast from polymer blends of natural origin (cellulose) or derived from the petrochemical industry (textile fibers). Regenerated cellulose membranes, both non-substituted such as Cuprophan and substituted such as Hemophan or di- and triacetate cellulose are hydrophilic. The synthetic polymer membranes may be either hydrophilic (Polyetherpolycarbonate, PC; Ethylvinyl alcohol, EVAL) or hydrophobic (Polysulfone, PS; Polyamide, PA; Polymethylmethacrylate, PMMA; Polyacrylonitrile, PAN).

> The hydrophobic membranes adsorb proteins, are more porous and have the highest ultrafiltration coefficients.

Permeability characteristics

Dialysis membranes are characterized by their resistance to solute diffusion, hydraulic permeability and sieving coefficient.

Table 4–1 lists current dialysis membranes with indications of their respective hydraulic permeability coefficient (Kf) and sieving coefficient (SC) for various solutes. A dramatic decrease in hydraulic permeability is seen in most of membranes when tested with protein-containing solutions, such as plasma, due to protein-material interaction.

> In high flux membranes, the decrease in membrane resistance is greater for high MW solutes than for low MW solutes.

TABLE 4-1. Hydraulic permeability and sieving coefficients of selected dialysis membranes. Glomerular basement membrane (GBM) characteristics are shown for comparison

Membrane	Hydraulic permeability (ml/hr.m^2.mmHg)		Sieving coefficient		
	Aqueous solution	Protein solution	Inulin (5200 D)	B2-m (11800 D)	Albumin (69000 D)
CDA (Althin)	36	16	0.90	0.70	0.1
CTA (Nipro)	60	16	1.00	0.90	0.01
PAN (Asahi)	ND	22	0.95	0.60	0.01
AN69 (Hospal)	50	30	1.00	0.65	0.001
PS (Fresenius)	170	40	0.99	0.60	0.001
EVAL (Kuraray)	14	8	1.00	0.63	0.04
PMMA (Toray)	70	13	0.75	0.00	ND
Diaphan (Enka)	80	ND	0.99	0.60	0.05
PA (Gambro)	260	35	1.00	0.65	0.001
GBM		200	1.00	0.95	0.01

CDA: cellulose diacetate; CTA: cellulose triacetate; PAN: polyacrylonitrile; AN69: acrylonitrile and sodium methallyl sulfonate copolymer; PS: polysulfone; EVAL: ethylen and vinyl alcohol copolymer; PMMA: polymethylmethacrylate; Diaphan: substituted regenerated cellulose; PA: polyamide.

Dialysate delivery system

The dialysate delivery system provides dialysis fluid to the dialyzer in appropriate conditions of concentration, temperature, pressure and flow. Dialysate is prepared continuously proportioned on-line (Figure 4–2). Dialysate and extracorporeal blood circulation are monitored in the dialysis machine.

Dialysate preparation

Dialysate is prepared from salts of pharmaceutical grade diluted in treated water. Salt concentrates are provided in powder or liquid form. According to their aqueous solubility, concentration ratio may be 1/35 (acetate concentrate) or 1/20 (bicarbonate concentrate).

Acetate-containing dialysate is prepared from a single liquid concentrate whereas bicarbonate-containing dialysate is prepared from two liquid concentrates, one containing sodium bicarbonate with or without sodium chloride, the other containing all other dialysate constituents and small amounts of acetic acid (Table 4–2). The latter is used to maintain the pH of the final dialysis fluid at 7.1–7.6 to prevent precipitation of calcium and magnesium carbonate. Sodium bicarbonate liquid concentrate can be replaced by a cartridge containing sodium bicarbonate in powder form.

TABLE 4-2. Composition of usual acetate and bicarbonate dialysates

	Acetate Dialysate	Bicarbonate Dialysate		
		Acid Solution	Bicarbonate Solution	Final Solution
Sodium	143	80	60	140
Potassium	2.0	2.0		2.0
Calcium	1.75	1.75		1.75
Magnesium	0.75	0.75		0.75
Chloride	112	87	25	117
Bicarbonate			35	31
Acetate	38			4
Acetic acid		4		
Glucose		8.33		8.33

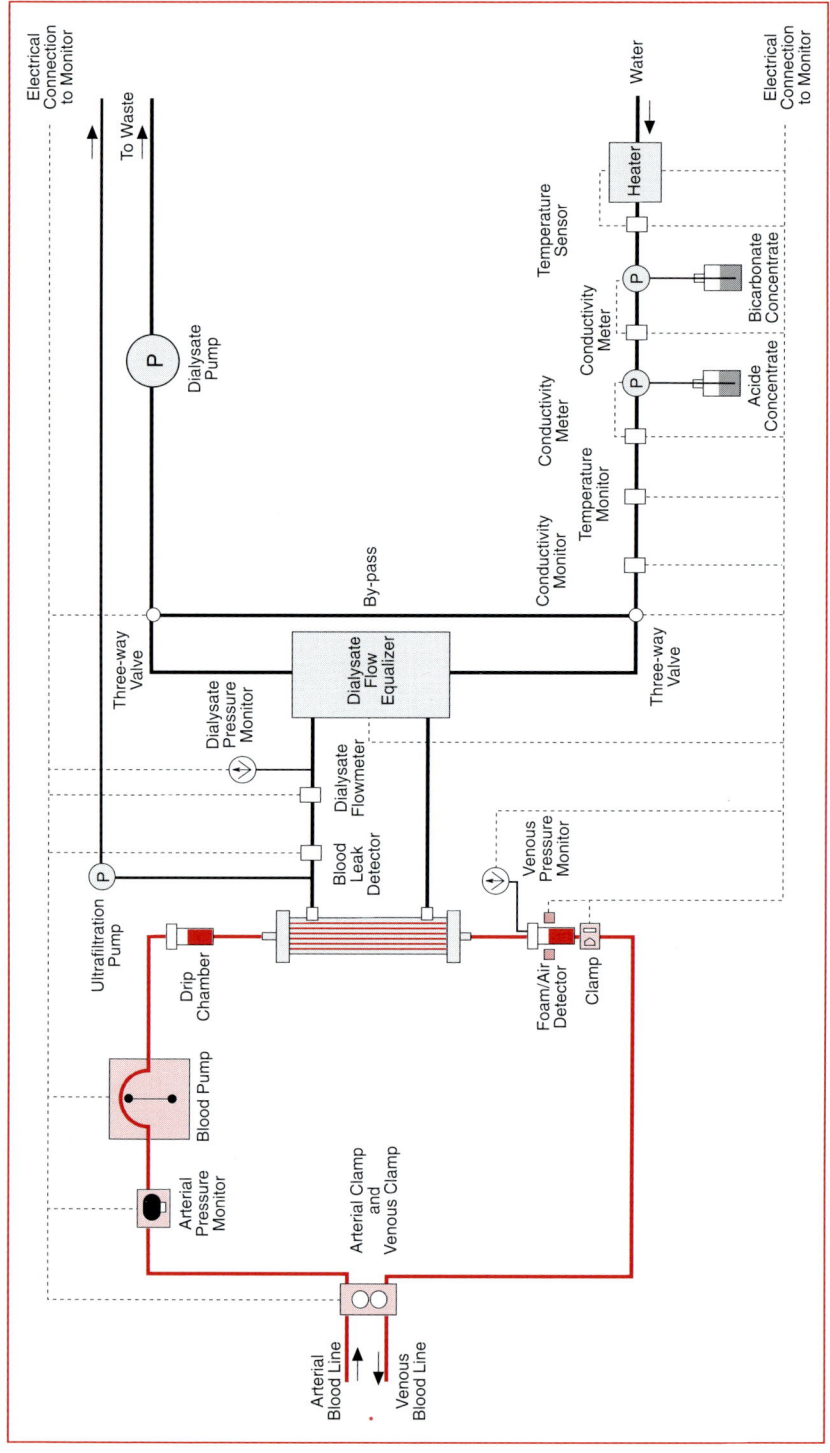

Figure 4-2: Diagram of blood (red) and dialysate (black) circuits with corresponding monitoring devices.

Monitoring

Monitors and alarms are deviced to control: (1) dialysate composition by conductimetry, dialysate temperature and pressure by specific sensors, dialysate flow rate by flowmeter or electromagnetic sensors, blood leak into the dialysate by photometry; (2) blood flow rate by calibrated blood pump, blood pressure by sensors, and air entering the blood line by control of blood level in the bubble trap; (3) proper use of various dialysate concentrates by pH-metry. Whenever these parameters are out of preset limits, the dialysate will be derived to by-pass, the blood pump will be stopped with blood lines clamped, and alarms will flash and sound. Monitors and alarms are designed to ensure patient's safety.

> Ultrafiltration monitoring depends upon the hydraulic permeability of the dialyzer used. To control and regulate ultrafiltration flow rate in high flux dialyzers, most dialysate delivery systems feature a dialysate flow-equalizer maintaining dialysate inflow and outflow rates equal.

Ultrafiltration flow rate is obtained by a volumetric pump which withdraws dialysate up- or downstream to dialysate flow. Alternative to a flow-equalizer is differential control of dialysate in- and outflow rates, using electromagnetic flowmeters or Coriolis's effect.

Hemodiafiltration monitor

An infusion pump coupled with the ultrafiltration pump infuses substitution fluid into the venous blood line to maintain fluid balance. Infusion rate is equal to the total ultrafiltration rate minus the fluid substraction rate prescribed for body weight loss. The composition of substitution fluid is similar to that of dialysate, except for the biofiltration mode where the substitution fluid is an isotonic sodium bicarbonate solution and the dialysis fluid, a base-free dialysate. Substitution fluid is sterile and nonpyrogenic, of pharmaceutical grade or produced on-line.

Computerized monitoring

Several dialysate delivery systems contain software programs included in the basic monitor or in an ancillary device for ultrafiltration and sodium dialysate concentration profiling based on sodium and water kinetics modeling, on-line blood density monitoring, automatic blood pressure monitoring, etc. These devices are intended to provide symptom-free dialysis and adequate removal of sodium and fluid, particularly in short dialysis. Newly developed on-line urea monitors allow to assess efficacy of urea extraction based on sequential dialysate sampling and urea concentration determination throughout dialysis sessions.

Disinfection of dialysate delivery system

The dialysate delivery system must be disinfected after each dialysis. The disinfection procedure should be performed according to the manufacturer's recommendations, which include the use of chemical agents such as formalin, chlorine, acetic acid, peracetic acid, or specific chemical brands prepared for this purpose, or heat. Disinfectant agents remain in the hydraulic circuits of the machine until the next dialysis when they will be rinsed out. Presence of residual disinfection agent in the dialysate should be carefully checked with an appropriate test such as the Hantzsch test or the Schiff reagent for formalin, or potassium iodide for chlorine and acetic acid.

> Periodic replacement of tubing of the dialysate circuit and the dialysate line is recommended to avoid the build-up of biofilm. Quick-connectors, which are prone to bacterial deposition and biofilm formation, should be disinfected separately and during at least for 24 h.

Dialysate composition

The dialysis fluid (or dialysate) is essentially an electrolyte solution with a composition close to that of normal extracellular fluid. Considerable variation has been advocated in both cation and anion composition in order to correct the abnormalities which develop between dialysis sessions. Table 4–2 shows the typical dialysate composition generally used.

Sodium

> Sodium is the major determinant of dialysate osmolality. Sodium concentration in the dialysate should at least equal that in plasma water in order to prevent an undesirable loss of sodium by diffusion. Indeed, hyponatric dialysate is associated with an increased incidence of hypotensive episodes, headache and muscle cramps.

Usually, a sodium dialysate concentration around 140 mmol/L is sufficient for the removal of 3–4 L of fluid with minimal dialysis-associated symptoms in almost all dialysis patients.

Potassium

A potassium dialysate concentration of 2 mEq/L is usually employed to remove potassium accumulated in the interdialytic period, during a dialysis session of 4 to 5-hr duration.

> However, a dialysate concentration of potassium up to 3, and even 4 mEq/L may be indicated when potassium depletion at the end of dialysis session provokes cardiac arrhythmia. This is particullaly true in elderly patients prone to cardiac instability.

Calcium

Calcium concentration in the dialysate fluid should be high enough to avoid a negative balance during dialysis. Since the diffusible fraction of calcium is approximately 60%, no appreciable diffusive transfer usually occurs with a dialysate calcium content of 3 mEq/L (1.5 mmol/L or 60 mg/L), although some calcium is lost in the ultrafiltrate. Therefore, dialysate calcium concentrations of 3.25 to 3.5 mEq/L (1.63 to 1.75 mmol/L or 65 to 70 mg/L) may be preferred to avoid a negative calcium balance.

Acetate

Because bicarbonate precipitates in the presence of calcium and magnesium ions, substitution of its precursor sodium acetate was proposed as an alternative.

In dialysis patients, the maximum acetate utilization rate is estimated to be 3.0–3.5 mmol/kg/hr.

> When using high-efficiency dialyzers, the transfer rate of acetate from the dialysate may exceed liver metabolic capacity thus resulting in hyperacetatemia. High acetate level has been implicated as a risk factor in dialysis-associated symptoms such as hypotension, muscles cramps, headache, nausea and vomiting.

However, standard acetate dialysate has the advantage of simpler proportioning devices and a large proportion of ambulatory chronic dialysis patients do well on acetate dialysis. The recommended dialysate concentration of acetate is 35 mEq/L.

Bicarbonate

Bicarbonate, as a base repletion agent in dialysis fluid, provides a more physiologic correction of metabolic acidosis than does acetate. In contrast to acetate dialysis, blood bicarbonate concentration and pH rise gradually during dialysis and the postdialysis increase is avoided. This results in less dialysis-associated symptomatology and improved patient well-being.

Usually, liquid bicarbonate concentrate is supplied to provide a final concentration in dialysate of 26 to 36 mmol/L, taking into account the amount of sodium bicarbonate consumed by acetic acid for the generation of carbon dioxide.

> Bicarbonate-buffered dialysate should be preferred in critically ill patients and in those with adverse reactions related to acetate, especially hemodynamic instability. In high-efficiency dialysis, bicarbonate buffer is mandatory.

Magnesium

Hypermagnesemia may result in disordered atrioventricular and intraventricular conduction, and nervous system depression. Chronic hypermagnesemia may play a role in renal bone disease and soft tissue calcification. The concentration commonly used is 0.5–0.75 mmol/L (1–1.5 mEq/L).

Chloride

The concentration of chloride anions is equal to the total concentration of cations (sodium being the preponderant one) minus the concentration of acetate or bicarbonate anion to maintain the electrochemical neutrality of the dialysate. The chloride concentration in dialysate currently varies between 105 and 120 mEq/L.

Glucose

> Hemodialysis is usually performed with a glucose-free dialysate. The amount of glucose transferred from blood to dialysate is estimated to be 25–30 g for each dialysis. The loss of glucose during dialysis may be responsible for dialysis-associated symptoms such as headache, nausea and post-dialysis fatigue.

Moreover, the loss of aminoacids is as high as 10 g per dialysis session performed with a glucose-free dialysate whereas the presence of glucose in dialysis fluid reduces this loss to 1–3 g. Aminoacid wasting together with increased protein catabolism stimulated by loss of glucose into the dialysate may result in a negative nitrogen balance. A dialysate glucose concentration of 1 to 2 g/L is recommended for diabetic and elderly patients.

> Patients without glucogenesis disorders and with adequate food intake available during dialysis usually tolerate well glucose-free dialysate.

Bicarbonate- and/or glucose-containing dialysates, which are media favoring bacterial growth and endotoxin production, introduce the risk of dialysate contamination. Rigorous disinfection technique associated with careful maintenance of machines and water treatment circuits is mandatory, and germ-free liquid concentrates should be used to limit these complications.

Water treatment

Tap water is unsuitable for dialysate preparation because its organic solute and mineral content is both variable and excessive, and should have detrimental effects to the patient due to the large quantities exchanged during an hemodialysis session.

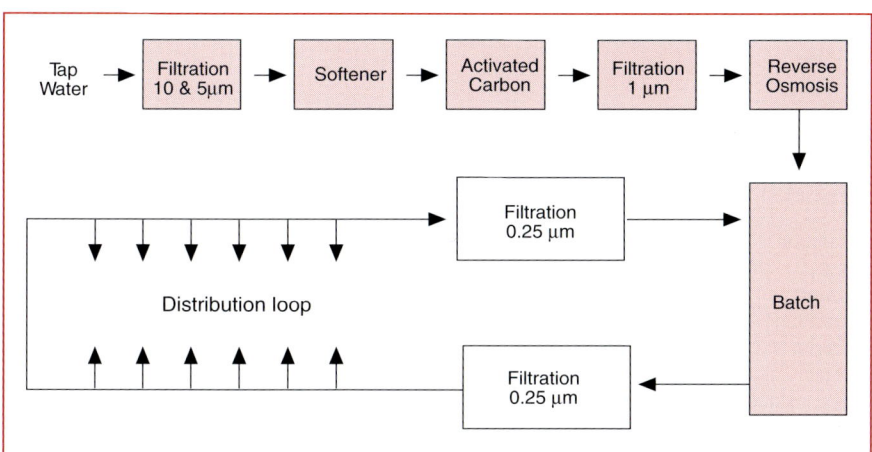

Figure 4-3: Schematic representation of the steps of water treatment for dialysis.

For the safety of the patients and to comply with the national standards, tap water must be treated. Maximum allowable levels of contaminants in water used for dialysate preparation are given in Table 4–3. The water treatment system is composed of filters to remove particulate material, a softener to remove calcium and magnesium, an activated charcoal filter to adsorb chlorine and organic matters, and a reverse osmosis device to remove most ions (Figure 4–3).

Insoluble particles between 5 and 10 μm can be efficiently collected by cartridge filters and particles down to 0.2 μm by membrane filters. Activated charcoal will adsorb organic matters, chloramines, chlorine, pyrogens and odor-producing material from water. Carbon filters are prone to bacterial infestation because of their porosity and affinity for organic matter. In a softener, the cation-exchange resin is in the sodium ion (Na^+) form. When hard water containing calcium and magnesium salts enters the resin bed, sodium will be exchanged with calcium and

TABLE 4-3. Maximum contaminant levels allowed in water used for dialysate preparation

Contaminant (mg/L)	Maximum level allowable	
	Association for the Advancement of Medical Instrumentation 1993	European Pharmacopea 1993
Calcium	2	2
Magnesium	4	2
Sodium	70	50
Potassium	8	2
Fluoride	0.2	0.2
Chlorine	0.5	0.1
Chloramines	0.1	–
Nitrate	2	2
Sulfate	100	50
Copper, Barium (each)	0.1	–
Zinc	0.1	0.1
Aluminum	0.01	0.01
Arsenic, Lead, Silver (each)	0.005	–
Cadmium	0.001	–
Chromium	0.014	–
Selenium	0.09	–
Mercury	0.0002	0.0014
Heavy metals	–	0.1
Chloride	–	50
Ammonia	–	0.2
Microbial count (CFU/ml)	200	100
Endotoxins (IU/ml)	ND	0.25

magnesium on an ion-equivalent basis. Saturation of the softener may result in massive release of calcium and aluminum. In reverse osmosis a semipermeable membrane with pressure process repels ions according to their valence and screens out organic particles while water is fed across the membrane. To obtain water having a very low ion content, a second reverse osmosis stage can be applied. Almost all particles of molecular weight over 200 Daltons are rejected, including bacteria, viruses and pyrogens.

> Special attention should be paid to the engineering and maintenance of the system to ensure the chemical and microbial quality of the treated water. Chemical monitoring should be performed at least annually and microbial monitoring monthly, with the possible exception of home treated patients. Careful periodic disinfection of the water treatment system is mandatory to obtain a germ-free and nonpyrogenic water.

5 BIO-COMPATIBILITY

Biocompatibility is defined as the ability of the dialysis system to perform without clinically significant adverse effects to the patient. Concepts of biocompatibility have changed with time. Formerly, evaluation of dialysis membranes and dialyzers for biocompatibility was restricted to toxicity and thrombogenicity of materials. Nowadays, great attention is focused on the interactions of blood with dialyzer components (membrane, casing and potting materials), residual sterilizing agents and dialysate components, and contamination of the dialysate by bacteria and lipopolysaccharide (LPS) endotoxins, which may result in clinical effects through complement activation and contact phase activation (Figure 5–1).

Activation of blood components

Complement activation

All surfaces foreign to blood activate human complement to some degree via the alternative pathway. As a result active fragments C3a, C5a and C5b-9 appear in blood leaving the dialyzer (Figure 5–2). The extent of complement activation and anaphylatoxins appearance in blood depends on the physico-chemical properties of the membrane.

> Unsubstituted cellulosic membranes are the most complement-activating membranes, due to the presence of numerous hydroxyl groups on the surface. Substituted cellulosic membranes, such as acetate membranes where hydroxyl groups of cellulose are replaced

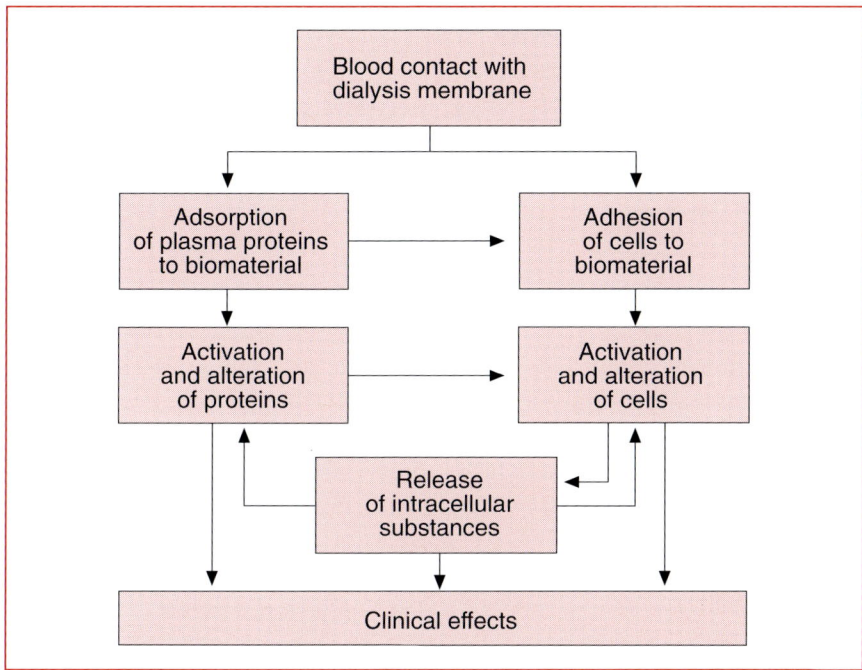

Figure 5-1: Multiple effects of blood-membrane contact [Adapted from Cheung AK. Membrane biocompatibility. In: Nissensson AR, Fine RN, Gentile DE (eds) Clinical Dialysis (2nd edition) East Norwalk (USA) Prentice Hall Intl, pp 69–96, 1990, with permission].

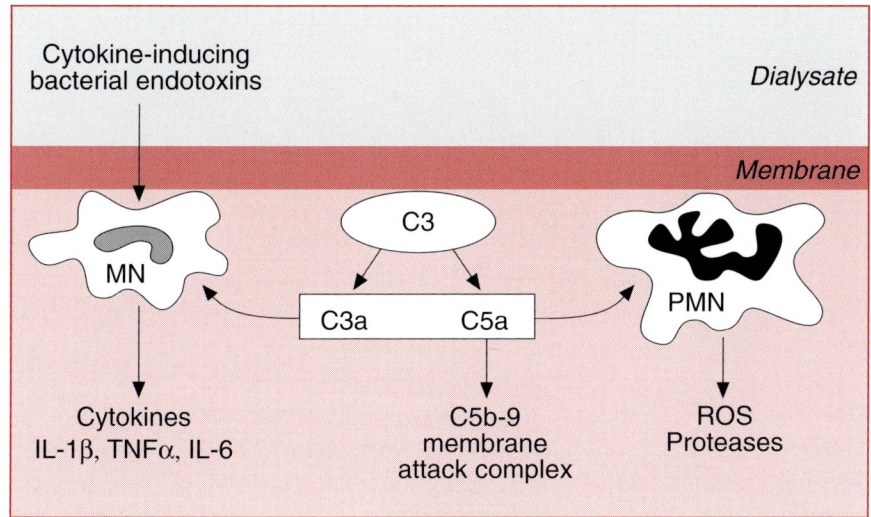

Figure 5-2: Mechanisms and consequences of complement activation.

> by acetate residues, provoke less activation of complement. The lowest complement activation is seen with synthetic membranes such as polyacrylonitrile (PAN), polysulfone (PS), polymethylmethacrylate (PMMA), polycarbonate (PC), polyamide (PA) or polyethylvinyl-alcohol (EVAL) where hydroxyl groups are not present in the chemical composition

Clinical consequences of complement activation

The activation of complement is maximum at 10–15 minutes but lasts up to at least 90 minutes after the start of dialysis with unsubstituted cellulosic membranes. During dialysis, complement activation provokes a profound but transient neutropenia which results from sequestration of the neutrophils in the pulmonary vascular bed (Figure 5–3).

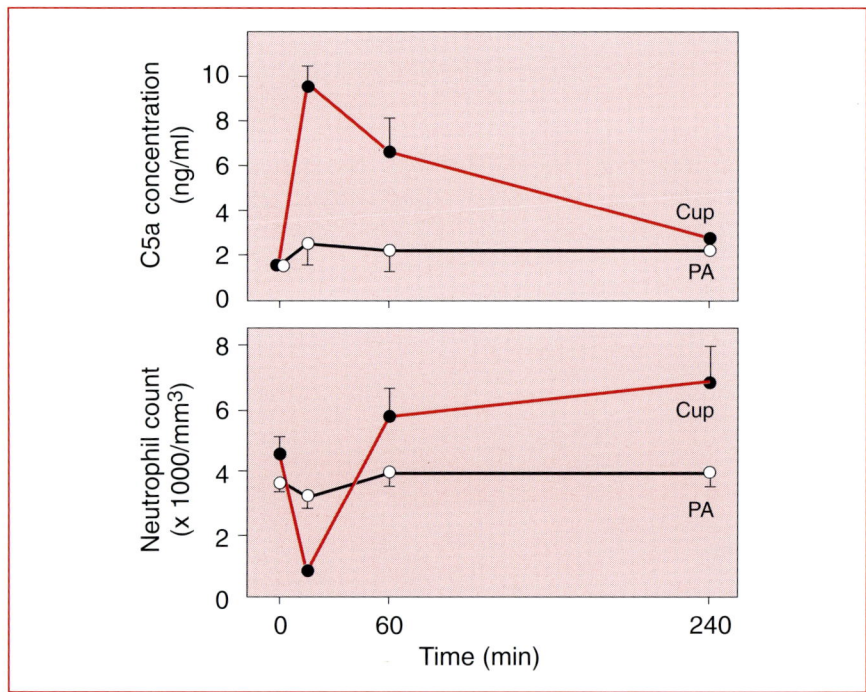

Figure 5-3: Time course of C5a release (upper panel) and of neutropenia (lower panel) during dialysis. Note the different effects of a complement activating (Cuprophan) and a biocompatible membrane (polyamide) [Adapted from Combe C et al. Am J Kidney Dis 24: 437–442, 1994, with permission].

> Fragment C5a is a potent biologically active agent capable of inducing anaphylaxis. Increased C5a plasma concentration is much lower with biocompatible membranes than with non-substituted cellulose membranes.

Other stimuli such as heparin, the sterilizing agent ethylene oxide (ETO), the anion acetate of the dialysate, and endotoxins transferred to the blood from a contaminated dialysate can also activate blood cells.

Reactive oxygen species (ROS) and proteases released by activated neutrophils, together with pro-inflammatory cytokines (namely IL-1β and TNFα) produced by activated monocytes may enhance β2-microglobulin release and polymerization, and endothelium damage. Following neutrophil activation, the down-regulation of opsonin receptors and adhesion molecules impairs phagocytic activity of PMNs, whereas deactivation of oxidase complex decreases their bactericidal capacity. Histamine and leukotrienes resulting from basophil activation can induce bronchoconstriction and vasodilation, and increased venous permeability. IL-1β and TNFα, synthesized and secreted by monocytes, can provoke hypotension and fever.

> The increase in plasma level of anaphylatoxins and proinflammatory mediators may be blunted when using high flux biocompatible membranes, due to the combined effect of adsorption onto and transfer across such membranes.

Activation of blood coagulation

Activation of the Hageman factor (Factor XII) due to the negative charges of dialysis membranes such as PAN membranes, when the pH of the priming fluid in blood circuit is lower than 7.4, can trigger the kallikrein cascade, resulting in excessive production of bradykinin. Because angiotensin-converting enzyme (ACE) inhibitors also inhibit bradykinin breakdown, anaphylactoid reactions can be seen in patients dialyzed with PAN membranes and inadvertently overtreated with ACE inhibitors (Figure 5–4).

Acute anaphylactoid reactions

Some patients appear to activate the complement pathway more vigorously than others when receiving dialysis with new non-substituded cellulosic

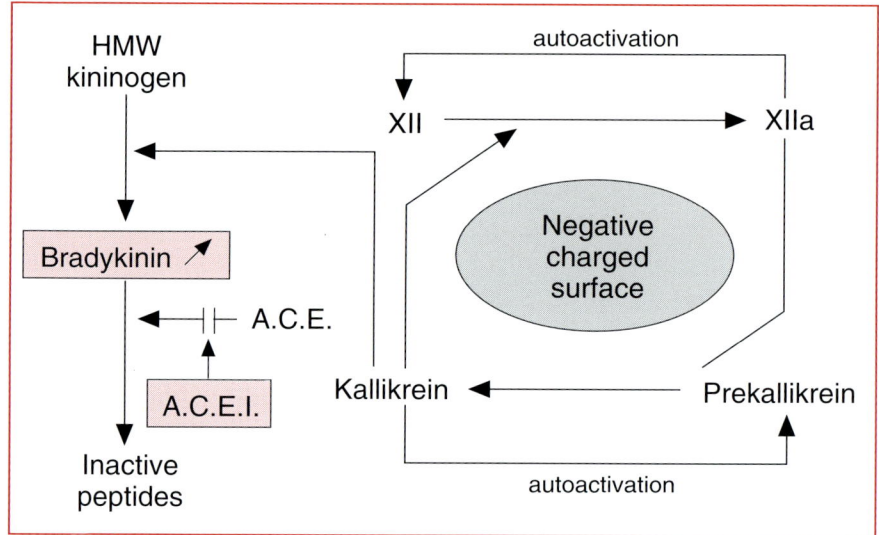

Figure 5-4: Mechanism of anaphylactoid reactions induced by negatively charged membranes in patients taking ACE-inhibitors.

membranes. The onset of reactions is usually immediate or within the first 5 min of dialysis and such acute reactions are identified as "first-use syndrome", since reprocessed cellulosic membranes have an attenuated ability to activate complement.

Reactions are typical of anaphylaxis and can be severe (up to respiratory and cardiac arrest). However, the etiology of early acute dialysis reactions also includes ETO hypersensitivity, endotoxin transfer from contaminated dialysate, excess of bradykinin due to concomitant use of ACE inhibitors and PAN membranes.

Major anaphylactoid reactions are uncommon. Flushed skin, chest pain, back pain and shortness of breath are the most frequently observed adverse symptoms.

Immediate treatment consists of stopping dialysis without returning the blood, together with intravenous administration of corticosteroids and respiratory support if needed.

> Prevention of the anaphylactoid reaction includes dialyzer rinsing with a large amount of fluid (2 to 3 liters) to remove leachables toxic compounds. If ETO is suspected, change to a gamma-ray or steam sterilized dialyzer. For patients dialyzed with PAN membranes and taking ACE inhibitors, discontinue ACE inhibitor therapy or change the mode of priming. When clinical manifestations suggest a pyro-

> genic reaction or bacteremia, verify water treatment and dialysate for bacteria and endotoxin levels.

Long-term consequences of bioincompatibility

In addition to its acute effects, activation of immunocompetent cells during hemodialysis sessions results in long-term deleterious effects.

> Stimuli that activate monocytes play a central role in dialysis-related bioincompatibility, by inducing a chronic inflammatory state mediated by enhanced secretion of inflammatory cytokines. Such disorders may favor dialysis-related amyloidosis, increased susceptibility to infections and increased muscle protein catabolism.

Bioincompatibility of dialysis membranes may participate in the development of β2-microglobulin (β2-m) amyloidosis. Unsubstituted cellulosic membranes may induce increased synthesis and release of β2-m by monocytes, and release of proteases and reactive oxygen species (ROS) which could favor β2-microglobulin amyloid fibril formation. In addition, those membranes do not allow any removal of β2-m. Thus, the development of β2-microglobulin amyloidosis with the use of low-flux unsubstituted cellulosic membranes results from the combined effects of increased synthesis, lack of removal, and conditions that favor β2-microglobulin polymerization.

Bioincompatible membranes play an important role in enhanced susceptibility to infections. Dialysis with unsubstituted cellulosic membranes leads to an impaired ability to respond to phagocytic stimuli, due to defects in granulocyte chemotaxis and adherence.

Protein catabolism is enhanced in patients on dialysis with unsubstituted cellulosic membranes through monocyte activation, release of cytokines and their subsequent action on muscle cells. Bioincompatibility of membranes may thus contribute to malnutrition in dialysis patients.

> Bioincompatible membranes contribute in several ways to increase the long-term deleterious consequences of hemodialysis, such as b2-m amyloidosis, malnutrition, muscle catabolism and impaired resistance to infection, whereas recent, more biocompatible membranes contribute to lessen (or prevent) such consequences and should be preferred when cost is not a discriminant problem.

The optimal conditions to limit the inflammatory disorders induced by hemodialysis procedure are summarized in Figure 5–5.

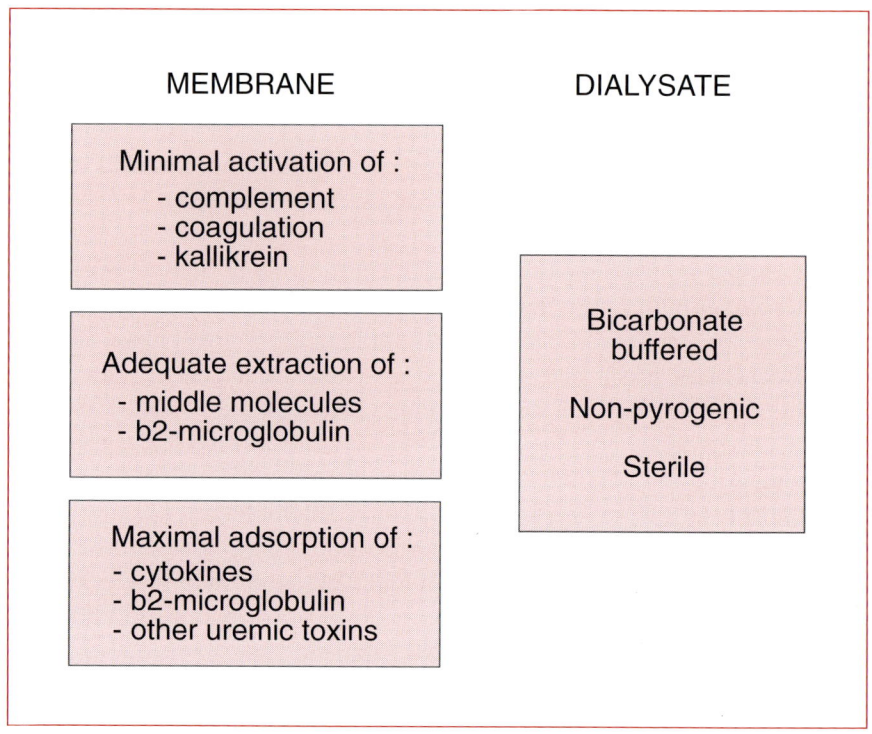

Figure 5-5: Optimal conditions to minimize hemodialysis-induced inflammatory disorders.

6 ADEQUACY OF HEMODIALYSIS, NUTRITION, AND DIALYSIS PRESCRIPTION

On a clinical basis, regular hemodialysis treatment may be considered adequate if the patient is in good general and nutritional condition, devoid of manifestations of uremic toxicity, and is fully rehabilitated. The main clinical criteria defining adequate dialysis are listed in Table 6–1. In the past decade, attempts have been made to define parameters predictive of dialysis adequacy, based on urea kinetic modeling, with mortality and morbidity as the main parameters to assess the therapeutic efficacy of long-term dialysis.

TABLE 6-1. Clinical criteria of adequate dialysis

Good general and nutritional condition
Normal blood pressure
Absence of symptomatic anemia, restored physical performance
Normal fluid, electrolyte and acid-base balance
Controle of phosphorus and calcium metabolism, and lack of osteodystrophy
Absence of other uremia-related complications
Personal, familial and professional rehabilitation
Fair quality of life

Quantification of dialysis efficacy

Urea kinetic modeling: The Kt/V concept

Using a 3-weekly dialysis session schedule, blood urea concentration has a discontinuous course, with a rapid fall during dialysis sessions and a progressive increase during the interdialytic period (Figure 6–1).

Blood urea concentration at the termination of a dialysis session (C_t) is

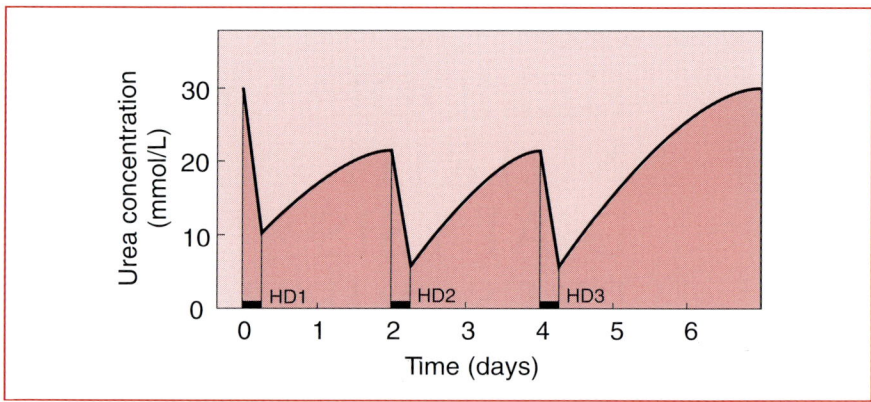

Figure 6-1: The discontinuous time course of serum urea concentration over one week with a thrice-weekly dialysis schedule.

related to its concentration at the start of the dialysis session (Co) according to the relation:

$$C_t = C_0 \cdot e^{-\frac{Kt}{V}}$$

where K is the urea clearance of the dialyzer, t is the effective duration of the dialysis session, and V is the diffusion volume of urea, i.e., the total body water space of the patient, approximately 58% of dry body weight.

The relation may be written as

$$\frac{C_t}{C_0} = e^{-\frac{Kt}{V}}$$

It results that

$$\frac{Kt}{V} = \text{Ln} \frac{C_0}{C_t}$$

> Thus, the dimensionless Kt/V index may be calculated from Co and Ct without knowledge of t, K or V. As an example, if pre- and post-dialysis urea concentrations for a mid-week session are 23 and 7 mmol/L, respectively, Kt/V = Log 3.3 = 1.29.

Urea extraction efficacy may be more simply expressed as the urea reduction ratio (URR), based on Co and Ct values, according to the relation:

$$URR = \frac{Co-Ct}{Co}$$

ADEQUACY OF HEMODIALYSIS, NUTRITION, AND DIALYSIS PRESCRIPTION

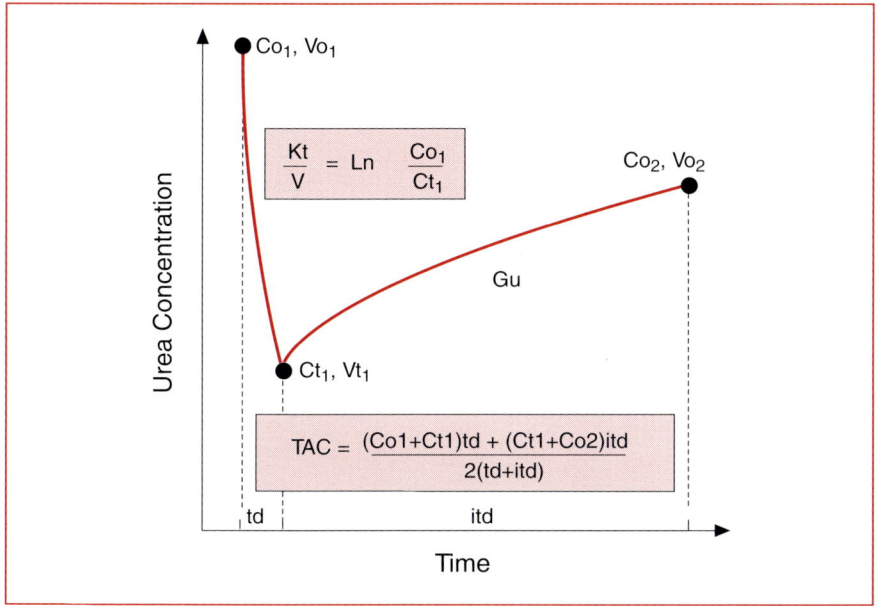

Figure 6-2: Parameters used to calculate the Kt/V_{urea} coefficient and the time-averaged concentration (TAC) of urea. Abbreviations are: td=time on dialysis, itd=interdialytic interval, Gu=urea generation rate, C and V=respectively serum concentration and distribution volume of urea at o1=start of the dialysis session, t1=end of the session, and o2=start of the next dialysis.

With the same example, URR = (23–7)/23 = 0.70

The time-averaged concentration (TAC) of urea may be calculated as indicated on Figure 6–2.

Correlations between Kt/V (urea) and outcome

Higher toxin removal should be expected to result in better clinical result. As a matter of fact, the National Cooperative Dialysis Study (NCDS) first provided evidence of a direct relationship between urea extraction and clinical outcome. Uremia-related morbidity was high at Kt/V values under 0.8, whereas it continuously decreased at Kt/V values rising from 0.9 to 1.5. In addition, Lowrie and coworkers recently demonstrated a close relationship between URR and mortality, URR values below 60% being associated with an increased death risk whereas values in the range of 65–70% or more were associated with the lowest mortality rate (Figure 6–3).

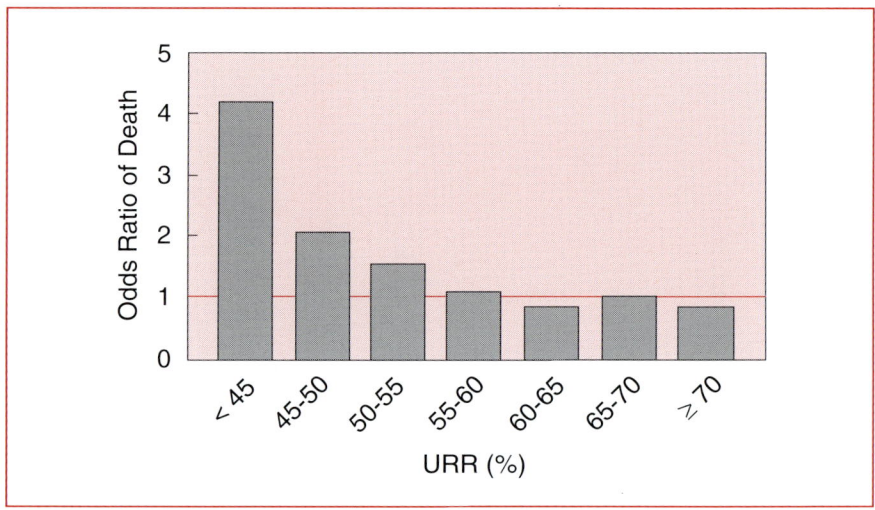

Figure 6-3: Relative risk of death as a function of urea reduction rate (URR). [Adapted from Lowrie EG. Am J Kidney Dis 24: 255–266, 1994, with permission].

Nutritional parameters of dialysis adequacy

Assessment of nutritional status: the PCR concept

Evaluation of nutritional status includes anthropometric and laboratory parameters. Some degree of protein and calorie malnutrition is observed in most hemodialysis patients as evidenced by reduced subcutaneous fat stores and muscle mass, low body mass index, and by suboptimal serum concentrations of albumin, prealbumin, transferrin and other visceral proteins. A lower than usual predialysis concentration of creatinine is suggestive of reduced muscle mass and undernutrition.

Mean values for pre-and post dialysis urea and creatinine concentrations in a selected group of patients of both sexes receiving 3 dialysis sessions of 4 hours each per week are given in Table 6–2.

A valuable marker of nutritional status is the protein catabolic rate (PCR) derived from urea kinetic studies. PCR (in g/kgBW/day) may be calculated as the sum of interdialytic urea generation (Gu) and of non-urea nitrogen (NUN) appearance during the same period. Assuming that 1 g urea results from the catabolism of 3.12 g of proteins, PCR may be calculated as follows

$$PCR = \frac{3.12\ [(C_{02} \times V_{02}) - (C_{t1} \times V_{t1})]}{itd} + NUN$$

TABLE 6-2. Mean predialysis (Pre) and postdialysis (Post) concentrations of urea and creatinine in a selected group of 10 female and 13 male patients in good general condition, receiving 3 dialyses of 4 hour each per week

	Urea (mmol/L)		Creatinine (µmol/L)	
	Males Pre/Post	Females Pre/Post	Males Pre/Post	Females Pre/Post
1 st session	29.2/9.2	27.0/7.4	950/399	874/336
2 nd session	24.0/8.0	22.0/60	872/378	813/304
3 rd session	23.9/7.9	20.9/5.8	817/360	724/276

where Co_2 and Vo_2 respectively are blood urea concentration and urea distribution volume at the start of the next dialysis session, Ct_1 and Vt_1 the same parameters at the end of the preceding dialysis session and itd, the interdialytic time duration (Figure 6–2). NUN value is about 30 mg/day, corresponding to $\approx$ 0.2 g/kgBW/day of proteins.

> In a stable patient, PCR closely corresponds to dietary protein intake (DPI) as assessed by dietary record.

Correlations between nutritional parameters and outcome

A number of studies suggest that malnutrition is an important risk factor for morbidity and mortality in dialysis patients. In the NCDS study, a PCR value less than 0.8 was associated with high morbidity, whereas mortality and need for hospitalization were lower when PCR was > 1. In addition, recent studies provided evidence that suboptimal serum albumin concentration (< 35 g/l) and predialysis plasma creatinine level (< 12.5 mg/dl, or $\approx$ 1100 µmol/l) are predictive of an increased death risk, as shown in Figure 6–4.

> Clearly, an adequate protein intake is of primary importance to prevent mortality and morbidity in the dialysis patient.

Interrelationship between URR and PCR

> An important message gained from analysis of the factors influencing survival is the close relationship between Kt/V urea (or URR) and PCR. In other words, protein intake by the patient largely (although not entirely) depends on dialysis adequacy.
> Underdialysis results in anorexia, decreased protein intake and low predialysis urea level, that may erroneously incite to lower the

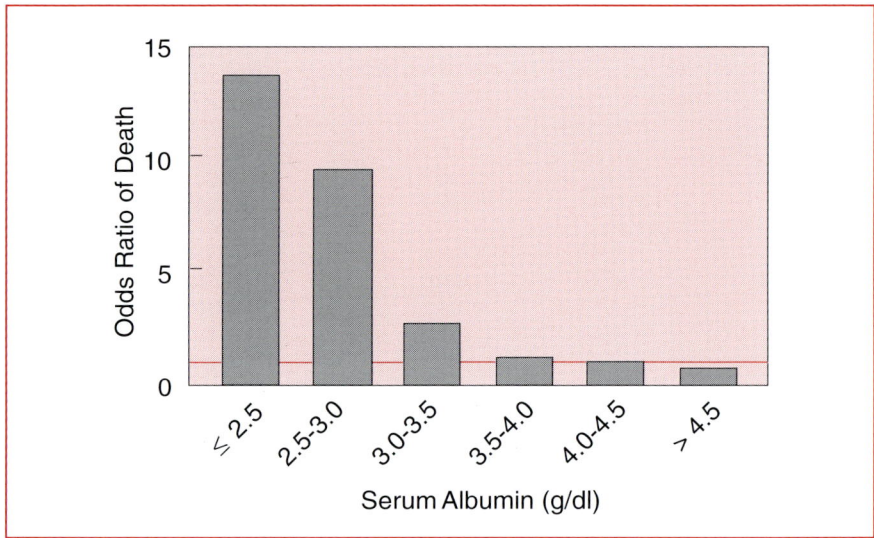

Figure 6-4: Relative risk of death as a function of serum albumin concentration. [Adapted from Lowrie EG. Am J Kidney Dis 24: 255–266, 1994, with permission].

> dialysis dose, therefore aggravating malnutrition in a vicious circle (Figure 6–5).

Only improving dialysis efficacy may restore appetite and adequate protein intake. In the NCDS study, patients with a Kt/V < 0.8 did not increase their protein intake in spite of active dietary counselling. Indeed, underdialysis results in accumulation of uremic toxins, both in the low and in the middle MW range, that directly provokes appetite loss especially for protein-containing food. However, malnutrition may be present even if dialysis is adequate, due to comorbid conditions.

Choice of adequate dialysis duration

Kt/V-based calculation of dialysis duration

One may theoretically calculate the minimum duration of hemodialysis (td) needed to achieve a given target Kt/V value, based on the urea clearance of the dialyzer (K) and the distribution volume of urea (V), usually estimated as 60% of body weight in males and 55% in females, using the formula

$$td\ (min) = \frac{V\ (ml) \times \text{desired}\ Kt/V}{K\ (ml/min)}$$

As an example, in a male patient of 70 kg, using a dialyzer with an urea clearance of 200 ml/min, a target Kt/V value of 1.2 should require a dialysis time calculated as follows:

$$td = \frac{(70{,}000 \times 0.6) \times 1.2}{200} = 252\ min\ (or\ 4.2\ hrs)$$

If a target Kt/V of 1 (usually considered adequate) is chosen, a td of 210 min (3.5 hours) should be judged adequate but would probably result in underdialysis.

Indeed, several factors contribute to overestimate Kt/V for a given prescribed td. First, effective hemodialysis duration is often shorter than prescribed. Second, dialyzer performances as determined on aqueous solutions overestimate by up to 20% the actual clearance of solutes achieved in clinical conditions; in addition, dialysis efficacy is furthermore reduced when significant recirculation occurs. Third, there is a "rebound" of Ct urea after the end of the dialysis session, due to incomplete equilibration between plasma and intracellular space, so that true final concentration is 10–15% higher than measured just at end of the dialysis session. This effect is especially significant in patients without residual renal function.

> Prescription of dialysis duration based on urea kinetics, with a target Kt/V value of 1, often results in an inadequately short td and, therefore, to lower than prescribed Kt/V and inadequate dialysis.

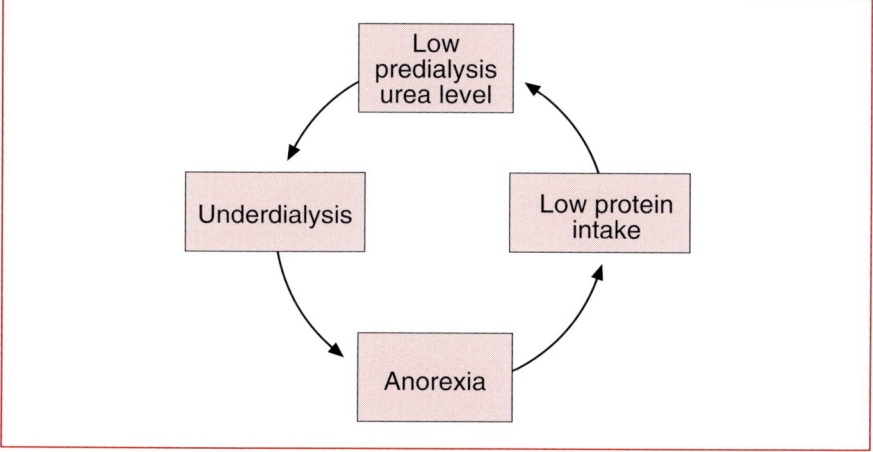

Figure 6-5: The vicious circle from underdialysis to undernutrition.

Adequate dialysis prescription

> Instead of using Kt/V to determine the minimum acceptable weekly dialysis duration, we propose to use Kt/V (or URR) to verify dialysis efficacy with an established, optimal td. Conditions ensuring optimal dialysis efficacy are listed in Table 6-3.

TABLE 6-3. Conditions ensuring optimal dialysis adequacy

Vascular access	: blood flow ≥ 300 ml/min during dialysis
Dialysis fluid	: bicarbonate buffer sodium concentration ≥ 142 mmol/l non pyrogenic (or sterile) dialysate flow ≥ 500 ml/min
Ultrafiltration	: permanent volumetric control
Dialyzer	: highly permeable, biocompatible membrane surface area ≥ 1 sqm (adapted to patient's body size) no reuse
Dose of dialysis	: Kt/V urea ≥ 1.2 Urea reduction rate ≥ 65%
Weekly dialysis time	: 12-15 hours (3 weekly sessions of 4-5 hours each)
Daily protein intake	: 1.1–1.2 g/kg BW (verified by dietary record)

> Consensus that a dialysis duration of 12 to 15 hours per week (divided into 3 sessions of 4 to 5 hours each) is the "gold standard" has progressively emerged during the past decade. Such a policy has been widely applied in European countries and in Japan for years and may largely contribute to the low overall mortality (5–8%/year) of hemodialysis patients in these countries.

By contrast, a higher mortality rate (up to 22%/year) has been reported in the USA where a shorter time on hemodialysis (about 9 hours/week) is usually applied. However, recent prospective studies in the USA clearly demonstrated that increasing effective dialysis time up to 4 hours or more per session resulted in a threefold decrease in mortality rate.

> Based on clinical experience, a Kt/V value of 1.2 and a URR value of 0.70 may be considered the recommended goals to achieve optimal urea extraction.

In addition to urea removal, hemodialysis should achieve sufficient extraction of middle MW toxins, including b2-microglobulin. High flux membranes improve dialysis extraction (by combined diffusion and convection) of such molecules. However, due to slow transfer from the intracellular to the extracellular space, middle molecules require a longer dialysis time than urea to be cleared.

> The need for optimal clearance of middle molecular weight uremic toxins is an additional reason to prohibit a dialysis duration shorter than 12 hours per week.

Dietary prescription to the hemodialysis patient

Adapted dietary prescription is an important component of the therapeutic strategy in dialysis patients.

Calorie-protein requirements

In healthy adults, a daily protein supply of 0.75 g/kg BW is considered a safe intake according to WHO recommendations. However, a higher protein supply is needed in hemodialysis patients in order to compensate for the loss of aminoacids and peptides into the dialysate, and the increased muscle protein breakdown induced by acidosis and by the catabolic effect of the dialysis procedure itself through generation of cytokines (especially with complement-activating membranes).

> A daily protein intake of 1 to 1.2 g/kg BW and a daily energy intake of 30 to 35 Kcal/kg BW are recommended to the hemodialysis patient. Such goals are often difficult to achieve, especially in older patients. Even if adequate dialysis is provided, a number of factors contribute to increased catabolism and malnutrition in dialysis patients, including metabolic acidosis, secondary hyperparathyroidism, anemia, infection, depression, loneliness or social problems.

Nutrition in dialysis patients is not only related to the balance between protein intake and removal of waste products, but also is dependent on the metabolic, hormonal and psychological disorders associated with uremia.

> Periodic assessment of nutrient intake by a skilled dietician is of primary importance to validate assumptions provided by PCR, to identify possible causes of reduced intake and to help the patient restore adequate nutrition.

Sodium and water intake

All water and sodium ingested in excess of the quantity excreted through residual diuresis during the interdialytic interval has to be eliminated by means of ultrafiltration within the duration of a dialysis session. Therefore, daily fluid intake should be reasonably limited to 0.7-1 liter/day above residual urine volume, and salt intake to 4-6 g/day, with addition of 2-4 g/day sodium bicarbonate to compensate for metabolic acidosis. Higher fluid intake should provoke an excessive weight gain, requiring a high ultrafiltration rate that may result in poor hemodynamic tolerance of dialysis sessions.

Nutritional prescription

Individualized dietary prescription must take into account all aspects that interfere with nutritional status.

Principles of dietary prescription in the hemodialysis patient are listed in Table 6-4. At least half of proteins ingested should be of high biologic value (i.e., containing the optimal proportion of essential amino acids), mainly supplied by meats and other animal products. Lipid intake should

TABLE 6-4. Dietary prescription for the hemodialysis patient

Protein intake	:	1.1–1.2 g/kg BW/day ($\geq$ 50% in the form of high biologic value proteins)
Energy supply	:	30–35 Kcal/Kg BW/day (60% as carbohydrates, 30% as lipids)
Lipids	:	1/3 unsaturated 1/3 monounsaturated (olive, colza or sunflower oil) 1/3 polyunsaturated (fish)
Carbohydrate	:	slowly absorbed carbohydrates preferred
Salt	:	4–6 g/day
Fluid intake	:	0.7 to 1 l/day in addition to compensation for residual diuresis
Potassium	:	limited consumption of potassium-rich foods (fruits, vegetables, chocolate)

be composed of balanced proportions of unsaturated, mono- and polyunsaturated fats, in order to prevent atherosclerosis. Correction of acidosis may require prudent supplementation with sodium bicarbonate. Calcium supplements (carbonate or acetate) affording 1–2 grams of elemental calcium are usually needed.

Supplementation with hydrosoluble vitamins is recommended to hemodialysis patients, as indicated in Table 6–5. Of note, OTC multivitamin preparations should not been used in uremic patients, because they contain vitamin A (in excess in such patients) and vitamin D2 (calcitriol should be used instead and the dosage adjusted individually). Special preparations formulated for uremic patients are available. In addition, folic acid supplementation at pharmacologic doses (2 to 5 mg/day) should be advisable because it has recently been shown to substantially reduce hyperhomocysteinemia, an atherogenic factor.

TABLE 6-5. Recommended vitamin supplementation for chronic hemodialysis patients

Vitamins	Daily supplement
Ascorbic acid (Vit C)	60 mg
Thiamin (Vit B1)	1.5 mg
Riboflavin (Vit B2)	1.7 mg
Pyridoxin (Vit B6)	10 mg
Cobalamin (Vit B12)	6 mcg
Folic acid	1 mg
Niacin	20 mg
Biotin	0.3 mg
Pantothenic acid	10 mg
Vitamin A	0
Vitamin D	Prescribe separately according to individual requirements

In profoundly anorectic, severely malnourished patients, temporary nutritional supplementation by gastric feeding and/or intradialytic infusion of aminoacids and lipids may be required.

Integrated dialysis prescription

Treating the dialysis patient is not just providing adequate removal of uremic toxins and sufficient nutrition. The nephrologist has to take care of the entire spectrum of clinical manifestations of uremic toxicity, in order to reduce mortality and morbidity, and to provide the best possible quality of life to the dialysis patient.

Figure 6–6 schematically depicts the clinical and biochemical components of uremic toxicity and their response to hemodialysis. Only a few of them (mainly removal of waste products and hydro-electrolytic balance) may be controlled by the hemodialysis procedure itself, whereas many clinically important deleterious consequences of the uremic state are not amendable by hemodialysis, but require specific therapeutic interventions, as discussed in the following chapters.

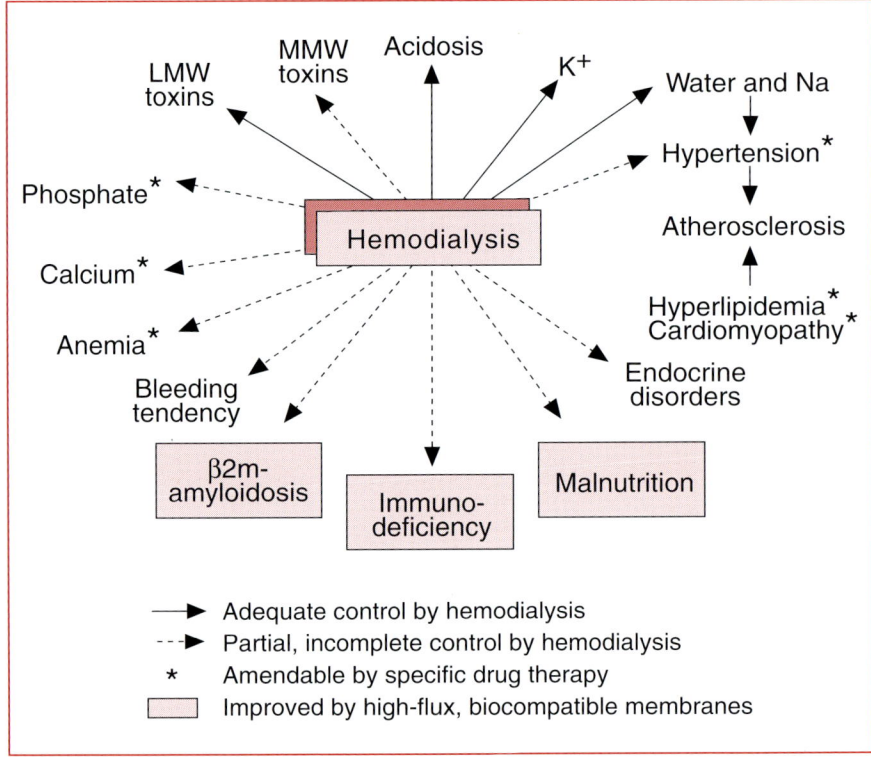

Figure 6-6: Schematic representation of the spectrum of uremic disorders with the respective effects of hemodialysis and associated therapy. [Adapted from Valderrabano F. Nefrologia, 14 (Suppl. 2): 2–13, 1994, with permission].

7 MANAGEMENT OF THE DIALYSIS PATIENT

Managing patients on regular hemodialysis treatment comprises monitoring of the dialysis sessions to prevent intradialytic hazards, and regular long-term surveillance of the patient to prevent, or limit, clinical complications associated with uremia and/or bioincompatibility.

First hemodialysis session

> The very first dialysis is a distressing event for any patient and adequate psychological support should be provided. The first sessions require particular precautions. They should be preferably performed in an hospital facility.

Dialysis duration should be short, using a moderate blood and dialysate flow, in order to avoid a too abrupt decrease in urea concentration that would result in transient intracellular hypertonicity and cerebral edema, with headache and sometimes seizures, described as the dialysis disequilibrium syndrome. Even with this precaution, some nausea and headache may occur.

If marked hypocalcemia is present, an intravenous calcium infusion should be maintained during the first dialysis session to prevent convulsions favored by the concomitant correction of acidosis. Hypotensive drugs (especially vasodilators and negative inotropic drugs) should be progressively reduced in regard to the volume and sodium depletion achieved during the first weeks of dialysis.

Monitoring of later sessions

Later sessions are simpler and usually uneventful. Monitoring devices and alarms now provide nearly absolute safety to the patient.

> More than 1000 hemodialysis sessions are performed in a single patient over a seven year period, with a thrice weekly dialysis schedule. Therefore, constant alertness is needed at every session to avoid any technical hazard and provide full security.

The hemodialysis procedure will not be described in detail here, because of its concrete nature and possible technical differences among dialysis centers throughout the world. Only the main steps will be briefly described.

Vascular connexion

Vascular connexion is the first step. The "arterial" needle is inserted far distal from the "venous" one to avoid blood recirculation.

Single needle dialysis may be used as an alternative when two sufficiently separated puncture sites are not available, but this technique results in high recirculation. Therefore it should preferably be used as a temporary vascular access.

> Needle punctures should be performed under strict aseptic conditions after thorough cleaning and large disinfection of the skin at the puncture sites. Disposable gloves must be worn during the whole process, to prevent any bacterial or viral transmission.

Heparinization

Anticoagulation is needed to avoid blood clotting in the extracorporeal circuit. General discontinuous heparinization is still a widely employed technique. Usually 5000 IU sodium heparinate are injected into the arterial line immediately after its connection to the dialyzer, and 2500 IU are injected mid-dialysis. General continuous heparinization may be preferred, consisting of sodium heparinate infusion maintained at the rate of 1000 IU/hour, with or without priming with 5000 IU.

> In patients with hemorrhagic risk, low molecular weight heparins which inhibit Xa factor activity without altering bleeding or clotting time are recommended. Heparinization may be totally avoided by rinsing the extracorporeal blood circuit every 30 min with about 100

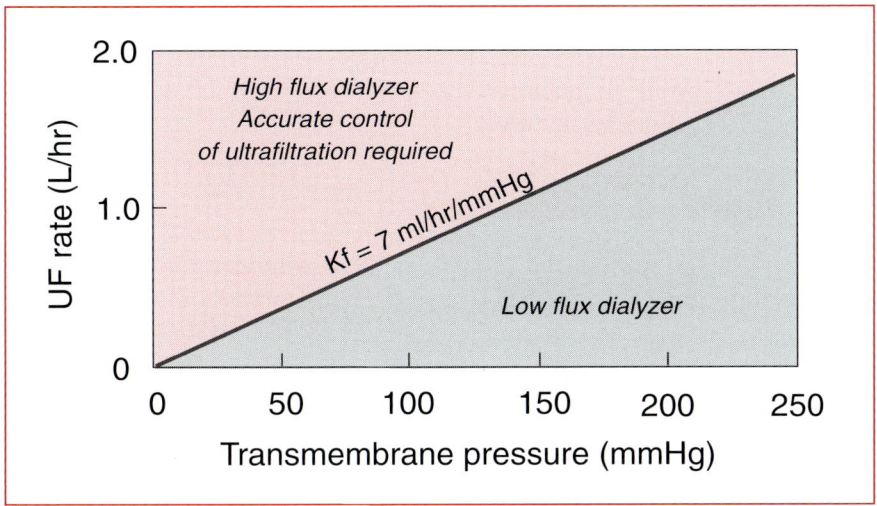

Figure 7-1: Relationship between ultrafiltration rate (UF) and transmembrane pressure shown for a dialyzer with a Kf of 7ml/hour/mmHg, measured in vitro, using an aqueous solution in the blood compartment.

ml saline, with adequate compensation by a proportional increase in ultrafiltration rate.

Fluid removal by ultrafiltration

The desired amount of fluid to be removed should be defined at the beginning of the session. It equals the sum of the body weight gain (difference between predialysis body weight and the desired "dry weight", i.e., the ideal end-dialysis weight at which the patient is normotensive), the fluid intake during dialysis and the volume of rinsing fluid used for restitution. The pressure gradient should be adjusted to achieve the desired fluid loss at a reasonable rate, adapted to the hemodynamic tolerance of the patient.

Ultrafiltration control devices allow to accurately set the prescribed ultrafiltration. Use of such devices is mandatory whenever high flux dialyzers are used, i.e., when Kf is greater than 7 ml/hr/mmHg (Figure 7–1).

Patient's activity and meals during hemodialysis

Activity is obviously limited to reading, writing, listing radio or looking at TV during dialysis sessions. Usually a meal prepared by the dietician is offered during hemodialysis. This contributes to patient's nutrition and allows to assess for appetite. Meat-containing meals should be avoided in older patients prone to postprandial splanchnic vasodilation which may result in symptomatic hypotension.

End of dialysis and blood restitution

At the end of the session, the arterial needle is withdrawn and clotting at the puncture site is achieved by gentle manual pressure and massage whereas the arterial line is connected to an isotonic saline solution to return the blood remaining in the dialyzer to the patient. When restitution is complete, the venous line is clamped, the venous needle is removed and hemostasis at the puncture point is achieved as above.

> Wearing gloves during blood restitution and compression of puncture sites is mandatory.

Clinical surveillance of the dialysis session

During each hemodialysis session blood pressure and heart rate should be measured and noted at least every hour. Pressure in the blood and in the dialysate lines, and ultrafiltration rate when using an ultrafiltration monitor should be checked regularly and adjusted if needed. Lying and standing blood pressure, together with body weight should be measured at start and at end of each session. All this information, and any eventual clinical or technical incident during the session should be recorded on the dialysis chart.

Technical hazards during hemodialysis sessions

Continuous monitoring of the blood and dialysate compartments should prevent all significant technical hazards, because any alarm triggers bypassing of dialysate and switchs off of the blood pump. The main hazards that may occur as a result of technical failures are indicated in Table 7–1.

A number of clinical manifestations can arise during dialysis sessions, the most frequent being hemodialysis-related hypotension and muscle cramps. Most can be prevented or alleviated by appropriate management.

TABLE 7-1. Technical hazards during hemodialysis sessions

Technical hazards	Clinical manifestations
Air entry in the blood circuit	Air embolism
Hypotonic dialysate	Massive hemolysis
Hypertonic dialysate	Hypernatremia, thirst, headache, pulmonary edema, seizures
Overheated dialysate	Hemolysis and clotting
Interchange of bicarbonate and acid concentrates	Severe alkalosis
Failure of softener used for water treatment ("hard water syndrome")	Acute hypercalcemia, headache, hypertension, seizures
Disconnection of the blood tubing	Hemorrhage, collapse

Hemodialysis-related hypotension

About 20 to 25% of hemodialysis patients suffer hypotension during dialysis sessions. Usually the symptoms are mild including malaise, yawning, dialysis discomfort and post-dialysis fatigue. The fall in blood pressure may aggravate cardiac ischemia manifested as angina or arrhythmia. In some cases, vascular collapse may occur requiring emergency measures. Such deleterious effects are especially harmful in older patients.

> The common mechanism underlying dialysis hypotension is the ruptured balance between cardiac output (which decreases due to loss of plasma volume) and failure to adequately increase peripheral vascular resistances (PVR). The key of the problem is an excessive contraction of the plasma volume, which occurs when the rate of removal of plasma water through ultrafiltration exceeds the refilling rate from the extravascular to the intravascular compartment.

A number of factors may contribute to such imbalance, as summarized in Figure 7–2. Prevention of dialysis hypotension requires methodic analysis of the factor(s) involved in the individual patient. The first measure is to readjust dry weight and dialysate sodium concentration in order to prevent a shift of water to the intracellular space.

> The use of bicarbonate buffered dialysate and of biocompatible membranes reduces vasodilation. Monitoring devices allowing continuous adjustment on targeted values of dialysate osmolality and ultrafiltration rate may considerably help to avoid dialysis hypotension.

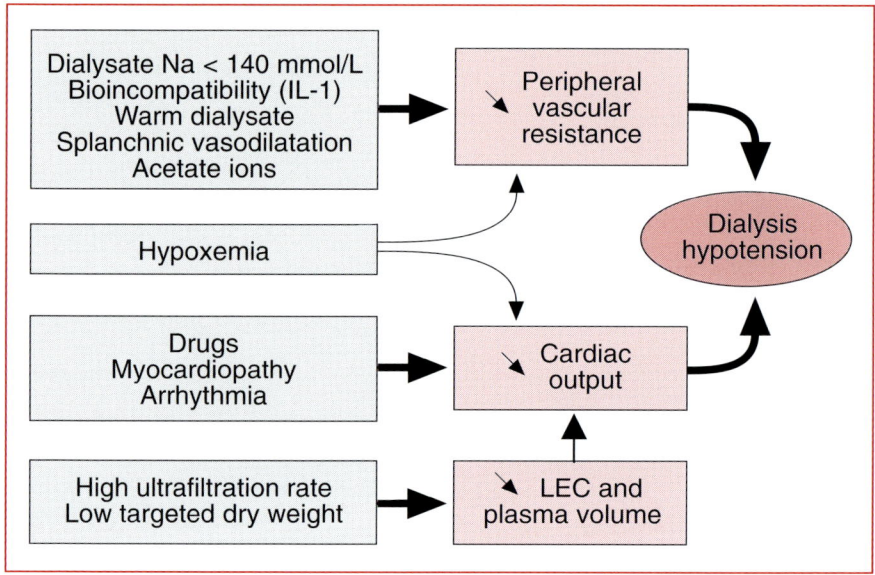

Figure 7-2: Main mechanisms involved in dialysis hypotension.

Other intradialytic complications

Muscle cramps result from extracellular fluid contraction due to rapid ultrafiltration or from inadequate sodium concentration. Administration of normal saline or of hypertonic saline may rapidly relieve pain.

Nausea and vomiting related to dialysis often occur in parallel with hypotension. If no hypotension is present, possible underlying gastrointestinal or hepatic problem should be sought.

Cardiac arrhythmia is not infrequent in hemodialysis patients. Ischemic heart disease and anemia are risk factors. Arrhythmia is favored by the rapid electrolyte changes (towards hypokalemia, hypomagnesemia and/or hypercalcemia) during dialysis sessions, and by the acetate-induced hypoxemia.

> Digitalis should best be avoided in hemodialysis patients. In patients at risk for arrhythmia, dialysate potassium concentration should be increased to 4 mmol/l, a precaution often advisable in elderly patients.

Chest pain appearing during hemodialysis may be due to angina, myocardial infarction or pericarditis, or associated with acute hemolysis or anaphylactoid reaction. In a patient with coronary stenosis, anginal episodes should be prevented by increasing hematocrit level, and using bicarbonate buffer and nitroglycerin.

Hemodialysis-associated hypoxemia is a frequent event when using non-substituted cellulosic membranes and acetate-buffered dialysate. The decrease in PaO_2 is modest (10–20% of baseline) and usually asymptomatic. Complement-activating membranes cause moderate early hypoxia (5 to 15 min after start of dialysis) in parallel with pulmonary leucocyte sequestration, whereas acetate-induced hypoxia is more severe, occurs later in the hemodialysis procedure (15 to 60 min), and adds to that resulting from membrane bioincompatibility.

> In patients with a precarious cardiopulmonary condition, hypoxemia may be symptomatic. Use of bicarbonate buffer, non-complement activating membranes and oxygen supply during dialysis should be recommended.

Interdialytic complications

Complications arising during the interdialytic period are mainly due to excess consumption of water and/or electrolytes (sodium and potassium).

Severe hyperkalemia (≥ 6 mmol/l) results from excessive intake of potassium-rich foods and is more likely to occur during week-ends which represent the longest interdialytic interval. In case of symptomatic hyperkalemia, treatment should combine immediate hemodialysis and oral or rectal administration of cationic ion-exchange resins.

Fluid and sodium overload may result in pulmonary edema, clinically manifested by cough and dyspnea. Immediate ultrafiltration will rapidly alleviate symptoms.

> Fluid overload may result from overestimation of the "dry weight" in a catabolic patient in whom muscle mass has decreased, especially during infectious episodes.

Modalities of hemodialysis treatment

Hemodialysis may be performed in dialysis centers, in limited or self-care facilities, or at home.

> Center dialysis, the most expensive modality, should be limited to patients having a compromised status or comorbid conditions requiring reinforced clinical surveillance.

Home dialysis is the optimal solution for cooperative and emotionally stable patients, with family support and adequate housing. Training usually takes about 2 months. Self-puncture of the vascular access is most often possible. Life conditions as well as the social or educational level of the patient appears of little effect on whether the training is successful whereas motivation of the patient and family are the main factors of success.

Self-care and limited-care dialysis are now valuable alternatives when either housing or family support do not permit home treatment.

> Both home dialysis and self-care dialysis lower the cost of dialysis therapy, while improving patient's autonomy and rehabilitation.

Long-term surveillance of the dialysis patient

In addition to routine surveillance during dialysis sessions, complete clinical examination together with laboratory tests should be performed on at least a three-monthly basis. Outpatient visits should assess the overall result of dialysis therapy in terms of adequacy and nutritional status; vascular access patency and cardiac tolerance; cardiovascular, neurological, osteoarticular, hematologic, hepatic, gastrointestinal and endocrine condition of the patient; social and professional status and psychological tolerance. Dry weight should be readjusted if needed.

Routine biochemistry is usually done once or twice monthly, in order to limit blood spoiling. Extensive laboratory examination should be performed at periodic intervals. The main parameters to be evaluated are indicated in Table 7–2.

TABLE 7-2. Regular surveillance of the hemodialysis patient

Total serum protein, serumalbumin

Serum cholesterol (total and HDL) and triglycerides

Serum transaminases (ALAT, ASAT), alkaline phosphatase, gamma-glutamyl transferase, CRP

Red blood cell count, hematocrit, hemoglobin, leukocyte count with differential cell count, platelets and reticulocyte count

Serum iron, iron binding capacity (transferrin), ferritin

Serology of hepatitis B and C viruses and of HIV

Intact PTH (1–84) serum concentration

Serum aluminum concentration

Electrocardiogram, echocardiography

Radiography of hands, skull, shoulders and neck

Chest X-ray

---

8 CARDIOVASCULAR AND NEUROLOGICAL PROBLEMS

Cardiac and vascular disease is the major cause of morbidity and mortality in dialysis patients. Hypertension, lipid disturbances and uremic toxicity play a key role in the pathogenesis of cardiovascular disorders. Overall, cardiac complications account for 40% of deaths in dialysis patients and up to 50% when adding cerebrovascular accidents (Figure 8–1).

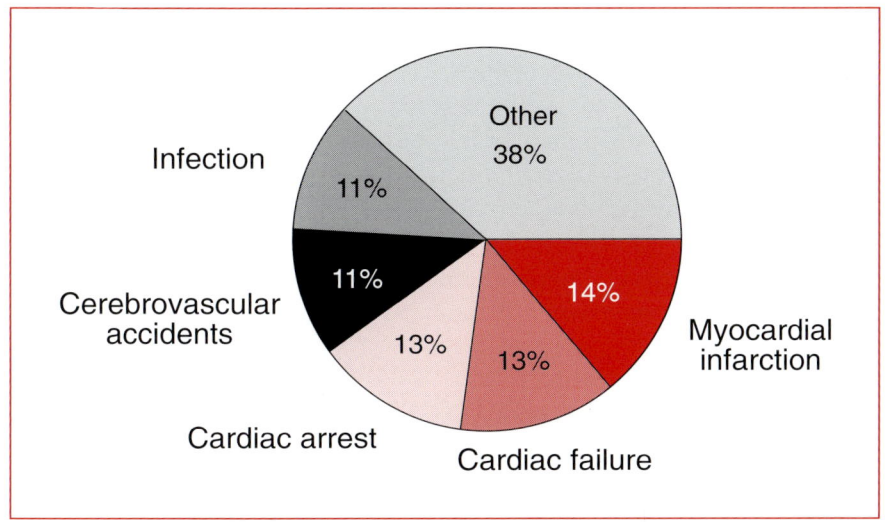

Figure 8-1: Contribution of cardiovascular complications to the mortality of dialysis patients. [Adapted from Raine AEG, Margreiter R, Brunner P et al. Report on management of renal failure in Europe XXII,1991. Nephrol Dial Transplant 7 (Suppl. 2): 7–35, 1992, with permission].

Hypertension

Hypertension is present in up to 70–80% of ESRD patients. Often the physiological nocturnal decline in blood pressure as shown by 24-hour recording is blunted, thus increasing heart work. Hypertension in dialysis patients is both volume-dependent, due to excessive sodium and water retention, and renin-dependent, due to chronic stimulation of the renin-aldosterone-angiotensin axis. In addition, increase in sympathetic nerve activity, endothelium-derived vasoconstrictor factors and/or blunted synthesis of nitric oxide, a potent endothelium-derived vasodilator, contribute to hypertension.

> Control of sodium and fluid overload by dialysis (with adequate restriction of sodium and fluid intake in the interdialytic periods) achieves normotension in more than half of patients.

However, if hypertension persists despite adjustment of dry weight, therapy with antihypertensive drugs is required in order to reduce morbidity and mortality related to hypertension. Antihypertensive drugs to be used in dialysis patients are the same as in therapy of essential hypertension, excepted for diuretics. The choice should take into account age and coexisting pathology, as well as the pharmacokinetics of the drugs, in order to avoid accumulation especially with some betablockers and angiotensin-converting enzyme inhibitors (ACEI). Hypertension rebound at the end of dialysis sessions should be prevented by judicious scheduling of administration time when dialyzable drugs are used. ACEI should be used cautiously in patients dialyzed on negatively charged membranes, in view of potential anaphylactoid reactions.

> With the combined effect of adequate fluid removal and anti-hypertensive therapy, blood pressure must be controlled in virtually all patients.

At the present time, "uncontrollable" hypertension is very rare and indications of bilateral nephrectomy for intractable hypertension in compliant patients have virtually disappeared. Failure to achieve control despite adequate therapy should alert to a possible superimposed cause of hypertension such as pheochromocytoma or adrenal adenoma.

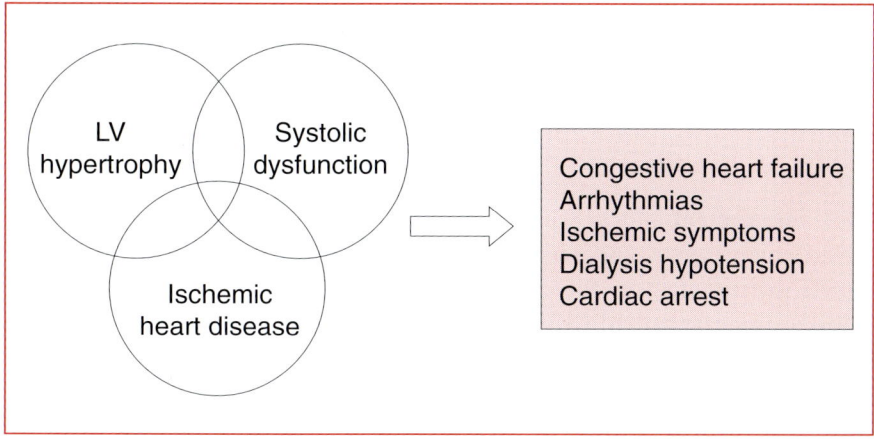

Figure 8-2: Manifestations of cardiac disease in ESRD patients. [Adapted from Harnett JD & Parfrey PS. Semin Nephrol 14: 245–252, 1994, with permission].

Cardiac dysfunction in uremia

Often cardiac disease is present long before the initiation of dialysis and tends to progress thereafter. Echocardiography is a major contribution to evaluating and following the cardiac status of the dialysis patient.

Cardiac dysfunction is multifactorial and may result from left ventricular hypertrophy, dilated cardiomyopathy and coronary artery disease, besides possible coexistent valvular disease and/or overfunctioning of AV fistula (Figure 8–2).

Mechanisms of cardiac dysfunction

Left ventricular hypertrophy (LVH) is the most frequent contributing mechanism, observed in more than 50% of patients prior to start of dialysis and in up to 66% on hemodialysis. LVH indicates diastolic dysfunction, with decreased LV compliance, so that a small increase in LV volume provokes a marked increase in pressure and may lead to pulmonary edema. The main risk factors are age, systolic hypertension and anemia.

Dilated cardiomyopathy is observed in nearly 20% of dialysis patients and indicates systolic dysfunction. The main risk factors, besides smoking, are hyperparathyroidism and uremic toxicity. Additional factors are excessive flow of AV fistula and chronic and repeated fluid overload.

Ischemic heart disease, related to atherosclerosis, may be present in up to 30% of patients. The main risk factors are hypertension, dyslipidemia, anemia and LVH. In all cases, diabetes, advanced age, high flux arteriovenous fistula, fluid overload and preexistent valvular disease act as additional risk factors

Clinical consequences and management

Such impairment of cardiac function results in congestive heart failure, arrhythmia, angina and hypotension during dialysis sessions. Potentially remediable risk factors for cardiac disease are summarized on Figure 8–3. Congestive heart failure requires strict volume control as a first therapeutic measure. The choice of pharmacologic agents may be guided by echocardiography. In the case of LVH with isolated diastolic dysfunction, ACEI and calcium channel blockers are the drugs of choice, whereas digoxin and inotropic drugs are contraindicated. In the case of dilated cardiomyopathy with systolic dysfunction and depressed left ventricle ejection fraction (< 40%), correction of hyperparathyroidism and ACEI are of interest.

> Of note, erythropoietin therapy reduces or normalizes LVH. Angina is also greatly relieved by correction of anemia.

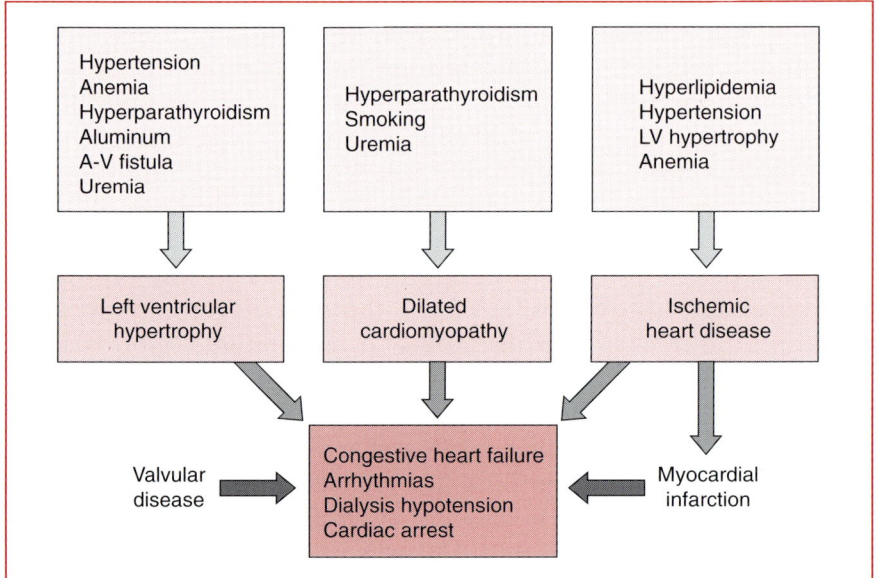

Figure 8-3: Potentially remediable risk factors of cardiac disease in dialysis patients. [Adapted from Parfrey PS & Harnett JD. Adv Nephrol 23: 311–330, 1994, with permission].

Atherosclerosis and coronaropathy

> Arterial atherosclerosis involving coronary, cerebral and peripheral arteries is observed more frequently in uremic patients, either dialyzed or not, than in normal age-matched subjects, thus justifying the term "accelerated atherosclerosis" proposed by Lindner and Scribner twenty years ago.

Factors of accelerated atherosclerosis

In the uremic patient, common risk factors (dyslipidemia, smoking, hypertension and age) and specific risk factors (anemia, hyperparathyroidism, aluminum intoxication, hyperhomocysteinemia, hyperfibrinemia, vitamin deficiency, arteriovenous shunt) add their deleterious effects to induce coronary artery lesions and ischemic heart disease. Myocardial infarction is the leading cause of death in ESRD patients and its incidence has not decreased in this population over time, by contrast to the general population. This suggests a role for factors specific to uremia. Older age and diabetes are additional risk factors.

Clinical expression and diagnostic procedures

Coronary artery disease is usually responsible for symptomatic ischemic heart disease in ESRD patients, and onset of angina pectoris frequently antedates initiation of dialysis. Coronary angiography evidences significant coronary occlusion in at least 75% of symptomatic patients. However, in about 25% of cases, ischemic symptoms without significant coronary narrowing may exist, thus suggesting nonatherosclerotic myocardial ischemia due to the combined effects of ventricular hypertrophy and anemia on coronary microcirculation. On the other hand, silent myocardial ischemia is frequent, especially in diabetics. Diagnostic procedures in ESRD patients are debated. Exercise ECG testing is often difficult to interpret because of the low effort tolerance of these patients. Thallium scintigraphy with dipyridamole stress testing improves predictive accur-acy.

> Coronary angiography is of major interest to evaluate the presence, degree, extent and thus potential curability of coronary stenosis. Indications of coronarography are increasing, especially as part of pretransplantation evaluation.

Osmotic concentration of contrast agents may produce pulmonary edema, which may be prevented by performing dialysis with sufficient fluid removal prior to catheterization. Using a small volume of low osmolality contrast media eliminates the need for rapid post-angiography dialysis.

Therapeutic management

Therapeutic strategy aimes at reducing the risk factors for heart disease, namely anemia, smoking and dyslipidemia, together with control of extracellular fluid overload, hypertension and LVH. Blood pressure control is of primary importance. Correction of anemia with erythropoietin improves angina, especially in patients in whom angina appears when hematocrit falls below a critical level.

> The use of bicarbonate in dialysis fluid, slow ultrafiltration, and reduced fluid accumulation in the interdialytic period contribute to better hemodynamic tolerance of dialysis sessions.

Long-acting nitrates are effective to reduce anginal symptoms during dialysis. Betablockers, calcium channel blockers, and/or ACEI are of value to reduce workload of the heart.

Coronary artery bypass grafting can be performed in dialysis patients with a short-term mortality rate now lower than 10% and appears to provide more sustained long-term results than does percutaneous transluminal coronary angioplasty, which however may be preferred in patients with very high surgical risk.

> In all cases it is important to treat preventively from the predialysis period by controlling hypertension, anemia, diet and major dyslipidemia, and prohibiting smoking.

Pericarditis

Symptomatic pericarditis is now a rare complication in ESRD patients, thanks to the generalized early initiation of dialysis. When occurring in the predialytic phase, uremic pericarditis is mainly observed in patients with marked nitrogen retention, hyperuricemia and massive fluid overload, and usually improves rapidly with initiation of dialysis.

> When arising in a patient on regular dialysis therapy, pericarditis is often associated with underdialysis usually due to problems of vascular access, and/or with an underlying infection or inflammatory

> state. Malnutrition and unrecognized fluid overload, possibly a reflection of inadequate dialysis, may be predisposing factors.

Chest pain and dyspnea alleviated by the upright position are the most frequent revealing symptoms. A pericardial friction rub is frequent, as more intense as pericardial fluid volume is less. On chest X-ray, cardiomegaly is nearly constant and pleural effusion is often associated. Echocardiography is the key to diagnosis. Anterior collection indicates a large effusion, which can progress to hemopericardium.

Recent-onset hypotensive episodes occurring early during dialysis sessions and thrombosis of vascular access alert to impending tamponade.

The first step in treatment is intensification of dialysis, with at least 5 sessions per week, with cautious and minimal anticoagulation. Prednisone or nonsteroidal antiinflammatory drugs (indomethacin) alleviate chest pain and control pericardial inflammation. If pericardial effusion persists after 7 to 10 days of intensive dialysis, or if hemodynamic evidence of tamponade appears, the pericardial effusion should be rapidly drained by means of subxiphoid percutaneous pericardiotomy with a pericardial catheter placed for some days, or by pericardiocentesis in the case of life-threatening tamponade.

Valvular heart disease

Preexistent, rheumatic valvular disease may coexist with uremic cardiomyopathy and markedly impairs prognosis.

> Secondary calcification of mitral and/or aortic valves is frequent in patients after a long duration of treatment by dialysis.

Hyperparathyroidism and/or high dose oral calcium supplementation are risk factors. Progression of calcified aortic stenosis requires surgical valve replacement. Acute endocarditis with valvular localization results from septic metastases after vascular access infection, and may oblige to surgical repair.

Uremic neurological involvement

Uremic encephalopathy

Uremic encephalopathy is now rare. This term describes functional alterations of the central nervous system that are part of advanced uremic syndrome. Manifestations are behavioral disorders: intellectual asthenia, decreased alertness, inability to maintain attention and to concentrate, irritability, anxiety, insomnia with somnolence during the daytime. Later appear disorientation, confusion and torpor. Neuromuscular disorders may occur in the form of cramps, tremulousness, asterixis and myoclonus. All these disorders rapidly and completely regress with dialysis, thus suggesting a role for dialyzable toxins.

> In fact, a large part of such disorders is due to anemia, as shown by the marked improvement following its correction.

Uremic polyneuropathy

Uremic polyneuropathy first manifests by sensory nerve alterations, in the form of paresthesias, burning feet, painful nocturnal muscular cramps, and restless legs syndrome. Motor disorders appear later, in parallel with impaired nerve conduction velocity. Clinic polyneuritis is now very rare and can be largely prevented by early initiation of dialysis. When appearing during regular dialysis therapy, it alerts to inadequate dialysis and/or undernutrition. Intensification of dialysis with highly permeable membranes should allow regression even if motor involvement is already present. Failure of healing neuropathy points to other etiologies such as poorly controlled diabetes or drug-induced neuropathy.

Iatrogenic manifestations

Since most drugs are poorly removed by dialysis, a number of drugs that are normally eliminated via the kidney accumulate in plasma and tissues of the dialysis patient. While their nephrotoxicity is of no consequence in dialysis patients, neurological and sensorial side-effects can occur. Especially, benzodiazepines, phenothiazines, long-life barbiturates, and metoclopramide may induce extrapyramidal contractures, muscular twitching and even seizures and coma.

Aluminum encephalopathy

Dialysis encephalopathy, or "dialysis dementia" is a severe complication of aluminum (Al) intoxication, resulting from the presence of excess Al in dialysis fluid and/or the use of oral Al hydroxyde as phosphate binder. Manifestations are dysarthria, myoclonus, seizures, and progressive dementia. Associated evidence of Al intoxication comes from concomitant microcytic hypochromic anemia without iron deficiency, and/or Al-associated osteomalacia.

> The best treatment of Al encephalopathy is preventive, by using calcium salts (except for citrate that can enhance intestinal absorption of Al) instead of Al-containing phosphate binders, and dialysate prepared with tested water containing less than 0.3 µmol/L Al.

Cerebrovascular accidents

Diagnosis of cerebrovascular accidents has gained considerably by computed tomographic scanning and magnetic resonance imaging. Hemorrhagic cerebrovascular accidents occur more frequently in hemodialyzed patients than in predialysis patients, suggesting a role for anticoagulation. Hypertension is a major risk factor. Incidence of cerebral hemorrhage appears especially high in Japanese patients, with a ten-year earlier incidence and a ten-times higher frequency than in the general population. Continuous ambulatory peritoneal dialysis should be substituted for some weeks for hemodialysis in order to avoid anticoagulation and to reduce the risk of exacerbating cerebral edema. The same is true in the case of cerebral infarction.

> Subdural hematoma may be secondary to excessive extracellular volume depletion aggravated by heparinization. It should be suspected in any patient developing headache, dizziness and vomiting which persist despite discontinuation of dialysis. Computed tomography is essential because rapid surgical drainage may be required.

9 IMMUNOLOGIC AND HEMATOLOGIC DISORDERS

Immune system dysregulation

Infection is still an important cause of morbidity and mortality in dialysis patients, and reflects the immunodeficiency state induced by uremia. In addition to increased susceptibility to bacterial infections, uremic patients exhibit abnormally prolonged survival of skin allografts, high incidence of malignant tumors, cutaneous anergy in delayed-type hypersensitivity and defective responsiveness to T-cell dependent antigens such as influenza and hepatitis B viruses. Factors implicated in immunodeficiency of dialysis patients are summarized in Table 9–1. However, in the past years, evidence has emerged that such a state of immunodeficiency paradoxically coexists with a state of preactivation of most immunocompetent cells.

> This dual disturbance of the immune system manifests from the early stage of renal failure, worsens with progression of renal disease and is accentuated rather than corrected by hemodialysis.

TABLE 9-1. Factors of immunodeficiency in uremia

Uremic toxins
Protein malnutrition
Trace metals deficiency (Zinc, Selenium)
Pyridoxin deficiency
Iron overload
Multiple blood transfusions

Immunodeficiency

Both humoral and cellular immunity are involved. As shown on Table 9–2 all immunocompetent cell types are affected.

Besides moderate lymphopenia, there is no significant imbalance in the CD4/CD8 T-lymphocyte ratio. T lymphocytes show decreased proliferative responses to antigens and mitogens and impaired production of interleukin-2 (IL-2) and interferon gamma (IFNγ), suggesting a deficiency in T helper-1 (Th-1) cells. Specific antibody responses of B cells are also depressed. This may result from impaired cooperation with Th-2 cells. Monocytes show indirect evidence of an impaired antigen-presenting capacity. These abnormalities explain the poor responses of uremic patients to pneumococcal, influenza and hepatitis B vaccines.

Phagocytic and bactericidal activities of polymorphonuclear neutrophils (PMN) are markedly impaired, resulting in decreased defense against pathogens. Finally, the activity of natural killer cells (NK) is also depressed, contributing to the higher incidence of malignant tumors.

TABLE 9-2. Dual dysregulation of immunocompetent cells in ESRD patients

Cells	Deficiency	Activation
T Lymphocytes	↓ Proliferative responses to mitogens ↓ IL-2 and IFNγ production	↑ IL-2R expression ↑ Plasma level of soluble IL-2R
B Lymphocytes	↓ Antibody responses	↑ Plasma level of soluble CD23
Monocytes	↓ Fc receptor-mediated response ↓ Antigen presentation	↑ Synthesis of proinflammatory ↑ cytokines (IL-1, TNFα and IL-6)
PMN	↓ Phagocytic, chemotatctic and bactericidal activities	↑ Generation of ROS and proteases ↑ Expression of adhesion molecules
NK cells	↓ Cytolytic activity towards tumoral cell lines	↑ Expression of CD56

Immunoactivation

In addition to the underlying state of immunoactivation due to uremia per se, blood passage through the dialysis circuit triggers a cellular activation mediated by generation of activated complement components following contact of blood with bioincompatible membranes and backfiltration of bacterial-derived endotoxins from the dialysate.

A massive production of reactive oxygen species (ROS) and of proteolytic enzymes by PMN coincides with the nadir of neutropenia. ROS and long-lived oxidants such as chloramines, together with proteases, favor structural changes of $\beta_2$microglobulin. The production of pro-inflammatory cytokines, especially IL-1, TNFα and IL-6 by activated monocytes is markedly increased and in imbalance with their natural inhibitors. Activation of T lymphocytes, through increased expression and release of IL-2 receptor contributes to decreased IL-2 bioavailability. Increased generation of soluble CD23 by activated B lymphocytes may also further enhance T cell activation (Figure 9–1).

The uremia-induced activation of immunocompetent cells, repeatedly exacerbated by dialysis sessions, results in a chronic inflammatory state which certainly contributes to late-occurring complications of long-term hemodialysis such as amyloid arthropathy and premature atherosclerosis.

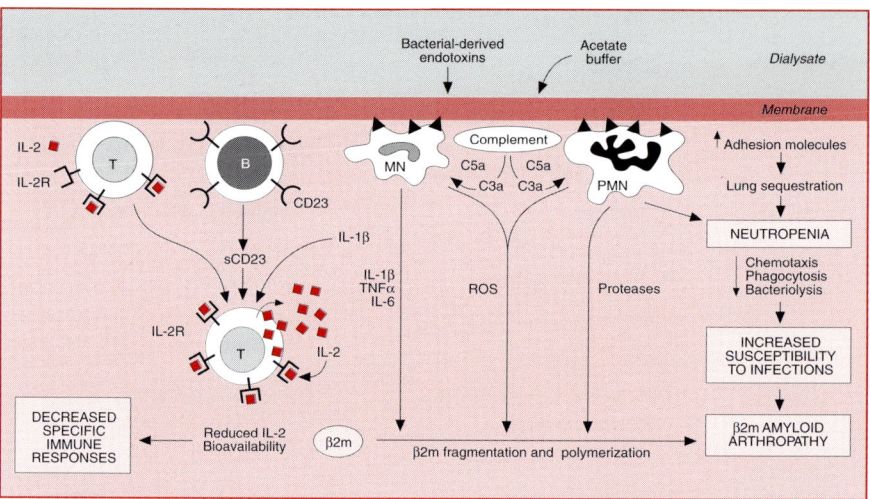

Figure 9-1: The effects of immunodepression and immunoactivation in ESRD patients.[Adapted from Descamps-Latscha B & Jungers P.Immunological aspects of end-stage renal disease. In: Jacobs C, Kjellstrand CM, Koch KM, Winchester JF (Eds). Replacement of Renal Function by Dialysis (Fourth edition), Kluwer Academic Publishers, Dordrecht-Boston, 1995, with permission].

Bacterial infections

The most frequent infections arising in dialysis patients are Staphylococcus aureus infections related to vascular access, and Escherichia coli infections originating from the genitourinary or gastrointestinal tract and from respiratory tract infections.

> Of note, opportunistic infections are not a frequent cause of morbidity in hemodialysis patients, because infections that arise electively in dialysis patients are most often due to micro-organisms against which mechanisms of defense mainly involve phagocytic processes.

Staphylococcal infections

Vascular access-related infections are virtually always due to S. aureus or S. epidermidis and may result in bacteremia, with the risk of microembolic localizations such as endocarditis, pulmonary embolism, cerebral or splenic abscesses, osteomyelitis and septic arthritis.

> Dialysis patients have a high prevalence of Staphylococcus aureus carriage in nose, throat and skin (up to 75%). Calcium mupirocin applied weekly in both nares is highly effective against such carriage.

Gram-negative organisms

Whereas the incidence of S. aureus bacteremias tends to decrease with time due to improved management of vascular access, incidence of E. coli bacteremias remains unabated. Such gram-negative bacteremias usually originate in the GI or the genitourinary tract and may exhibit an especially severe course in iron overloaded patients. The risk of urinary tract infection is increased in hemodialysis patients due to the very low urine output. An especially high incidence is observed in patients with a history of urolithiasis or with polycystic kidney disease. Tomodensitometry is useful to identify infected cysts. Isotopic scanning seems less accurate.

Gram-negative infections may also complicate colonic diverticulosis, liver cysts or biliary duct dilation in patients with polycystic kidney disease and may require surgery.

> Due to poor diffusion of antibiotics at infection sites, prolonged antimicrobial therapy is needed and nephrectomy may be required.

Unusual infections

> The incidence of tuberculosis is ten times higher in dialysis patients than in the general population. In most cases it consists of reactivation of prior infection and mainly involves extrapulmonary sites. Clinical presentation is atypical and poorly symptomatic, often arising in the form of prolonged fever, anorexia and weight loss.

Non-tuberculous mycobacteria have also been incriminated. Principal causes of long-duration fever in dialysis patients besides tuberculosis are given in Table 9–3.

Severe septicemic infections with Listeria monocytogenes or Yersinia enterolytica have been reported in dialysis patients with iron overload, and mucormycosis infection may complicate deferoxamine therapy, the latter acting as siderophore for Rhizopus strains.

TABLE 9-3. Causes of prolonged fever in long-term hemodialysis patients

Tuberculosis (pulmonary or extrapulmonary)
Malignancy (GI tract, other)
Reactivation of underlying systemic disease
Endocarditis
Viral hepatitis
Diverticulosis
Rejection or necrobiosis of kidney graft
Infection of vascular access
Thrombosis of arteriovenous fistula
Pericarditis
Nose, throat, ear, sinus or tooth infection
Pleural and/or pulmonary infection, either bacterial or viral
Urinary tract infection
Infection of hepatic or renal cysts in polycystic kidney disease

Viral hepatitis

> Hemodialysis has long been a high-risk environment for transmission of hepatitis B (HBV) and hepatitis C (HCV) viruses. Fortunately, significant therapeutic advances now allow progressive eradication of such infections, that are especially deleterious to patients candidates for kidney transplantation.

Hepatitis B

Unlike healthy subjects, uremic patients almost always have asymptomatic infection, that can only be detected by laboratory surveillance. Due to their inability to produce neutralizing titers of antibodies to the surface antigen of the virus (HBsAg), infected patients often remain chronic carriers of HBsAg with persistent viral replication, and thus constitute virus reservoirs that transmit infection to other patients and health care workers. Therefore, AgHBs positive patients must be dialyzed in separate rooms with reinforced disinfection of all dialysis equipment.

> Generalized active immunization with plasma-derived, and now with DNA-recombinant vaccines has considerably lowered the incidence of HBV infection in both staff and patients in dialysis centers. However, because of impaired responsiveness, uremic patients need reinforced vaccination protocols.

Additional vaccine injections (or a higher antigen dose) until a protective level (i.e., above 10 mIU/ml) of anti-HBs antibody is achieved are required. Booster injection at one year helps to increase anti-HBs titer, thus allowing more prolonged protection. Repeated anti-HBs titration and further boosters at appropriate intervals are needed. Hyporesponsive patients should be passively protected by regular injections of specific anti-HBs immunoglobulins.

> It is best to start vaccination long in advance of the predictable time of starting dialysis, for instance when serum creatinine is 300 μmol/l (3.3 mg/dl) whenever possible. Also, revaccination is recommended soon after kidney transplantation.

Hepatitis C

Until the nineties, the so-called non-A, non-B hepatitis, now identified as hepatitis C virus, was very frequent in dialysis units, due to transmission by blood. Thanks to serologic identification of HCV by ELISA tests allowing blood donor testing, blood transmission is now virtually precluded. At the same time, generalization of recombinant erythropoietin therapy has virtually suppressed the need for blood transfusion. As a result, the incidence of HCV infections is now very low, even if nosocomial transmission is still possible.

> In patients already infected, antiviral therapy with alfa-interferon may be indicated on the basis of the degree of virus replication assessed by PCR analysis and liver biopsy (preferably via transjugular route). It should be performed prior to kidney transplantation, because such antiviral therapy may induce graft rejection when administered to a transplant patient.

Because no vaccine against hepatitis C virus is available, prevention of HCV infection requires strict respect of the general precautions against bloodborne viral infections (Table 9–4). These precautions are also valuable in preventing nosocomial transmission of other viruses such as HBV and human immunodeficiency virus (HIV) as well.

TABLE 9-4. General precautions to prevent nosocomial transmission of viruses in hemodialysis units

1- Scrupulous cleaning and disinfetion of dialysis equipment and environmental surfaces before and after each dialysis session.
2- No sharing of articles between patients.
3- Change of gloves for each patient, especially for compression of the site of fistula puncture.
4- Regular screening for serum transaminase level.
5- Regular screening for HBV and HCV serologic markers.

Anemia and erythropoietin therapy

> Anemia is one of the major problems in ESRD patients because it considerably alters patient's quality of life. Fortunately, recombinant erythropoietin (r-HuEPO) therapy has recently led to efficient correction in anemia.

Mechanisms and consequences of anemia

The main factor contributing to uremia-associated anemia is inadequate production of erythropoietin by peritubular cells in response to local hypoxia, due to the reduced mass of functional parenchyma. Additional factors are reduced RBC survival due to guanidic compounds, chloramines, nitrites or splenic RBC sequestration, and impaired erythropoiesis due to iron deficiency, uremic toxins such as polyamines, vitamin deficiency (folic acid, vitamin B12), and blood losses due to GI or uterine bleeding, blood sampling and/or hemodialysis procedure itself.

IMMUNOLOGIC AND HEMATOLOGIC DISORDERS

Uremia-related anemia is usually normochromic and normocytic, with a decreased reticulocyte index. Macrocytic anemia should suggest vitamin B12 or folate deficiency.

> Appearance of hypochromic anemia with hyposideremia should alert to the possibility of occult GI bleeding, including colic neoplasia.

Anemia has major clinical consequences to the dialysis patient, because it is responsible for a permanent sensation of physical and mental fatigue, reduced exercice capacity, impaired cognitive functions, diminished libido and sexual activity, and lack of appetite. Anemia is also a major factor contributing to left ventricular hypertrophy, and to angina in patients with coronary disease, especially in the elderly.

Treatment of anemia

> The fundamental therapy, which has dramatically improved the quality of life of dialysis patients, is r-HuEPO. However, measures aimed at suppressing all sources of bleeding, and correcting iron and vitamin deficiency, are a prerequisite to r-HuEPO therapy (Table 9–5).

TABLE 9-5. Treatment of anemia in ESRD patients

1- Correction or prevention of iron deficiency
2- Adequate dialysis and nutrition
3- Correction of folate and/or Vit B12 deficiency
4- Treatment of gastrointestinal or uterine bleeding
5- r-HuEPO therapy

Because vigorous erythropoiesis requires increased iron availability, patients who initially have low ferritin level (< 100 µg/L) and low transferrin saturation (< 20%) should receive iron supplements. The iron need can be estimated by the following formula:

$$\text{Iron need (mg)} = 150 \times [\text{desired-present Hb (g/dl)}].$$

> r-HuEPO therapy is indicated whenever Hb level is under 8 g/dl, and/or if clinical symptoms such as angina or extreme fatigue are present even at an hematocrit level between 8 and 10 g/dl.

Management of EPO therapy

The starting dose of r-HuEPO is usually 50 units/kg BW thrice weekly by the intravenous route at the end of each dialysis session, in order to obtain a hemoglobin level of 10–11 g/dl at a slow rate. The maintenance dose is markedly lower, 50–120 units/kg BW per week. The subcutaneous route allows to decrease by about 30% the weekly dose and thus to decrease the high cost of therapy.

Possible causes of apparent resistance to r-HuEPO are listed in Table 9-6.

TABLE 9-6. Possible causes of hyporesponsiveness to erythropoietin therapy in dialysis patients

Iron deficiency
Infection or inflammation (overt or occult)
Aluminum intoxication
Severe hyperparathyroidism
Blood loss (GI tract, uterine)
Vitamin B12 and/or folate deficiency
Inadequate dialysis
Malignancy

> Benefits of r-HuEPO therapy are obvious. Patients recover a sense of well-being with improved physical and mental activity, appetite, libido and sexual activity and positive nitrogen balance. In addition, left ventricular hypertrophy regresses, and iron stores, when excessive, progressively decrease resulting in restoration of better immune defences. Suppressing the need for transfusions results in a lowered risk of viral transmission and iron overload.

Adverse effects and complications of r-HuEPO therapy may occur. Seizures are now very infrequent due to more progressive dosing. Hypertension is observed in about 20% of cases, and introduction or reinforcement of antihypertensive therapy, together with readjustement of dry weight may be needed. Increased blood viscosity as blood hemoglobin rises may favor thrombosis of vascular access (especially prosthetic devices) and decrease hemodialysis efficiency. In the latter case, increasing dialysis time and/or membrane surface area should allow to regain a correct Kt/V value. Due to improved appetite, potassium and phosphate intake often increase and may require correction.

> Thus, blood pressure, dry weight and dialysis parameters must be carefully monitored on EPO therapy.

Hemostasis disorders

Platelet dysfunction in uremics

In uremic patients, platelet count is usually normal, but platelet functions are impaired with prolonged bleeding time and defective platelet adhesiveness and aggregability. Accumulation of uremic toxins, especially guanidinosuccinic acid and phenolic compounds has been incriminated. Although these molecules are readily diffusible, adequate hemodialysis does not completely correct platelet dysfunction. Plasma levels of Von Willebrand factor (vWF) are high in uremics, but a defect in the vWF-platelet interaction may participate in the defective binding of platelets to subendothelial collagen. Lastly, anemia itself contributes to platelet dysfunction, and bleeding time is improved on r-HuEPO therapy.

Bleeding tendency

Clinically, increased bleeding tendency results in purpura, ecchymoses, epistaxis, prolonged bleeding from venipuncture sites and gastro-intestinal bleeding, due to frequent underlying pathology of GI tract. Treatment of the bleeding tendency implies adequate dialysis using reduced heparin dosage or low molecular weight heparins. r-HuEPO therapy has a beneficial effect.

When an immediate, transitory effect is needed for treatment of acute bleeding episodes, cryoprecipitate, a plasma derivative rich in vWF corrects bleeding time within 1 hour and its action lasts 24–36 hours. Desmopressin [1-deamino-8-D-arginine vasopressin], which induces the release of endogenous vWF from cell stores, can be administered intravenously or subcutaneously (0.3 µg/kg BW), or by the nasal route (3 µg/kg BW); its effects last for 6 to 8 hours. Conjugated estrogens, 0.6 mg/kg/day for five days by the IV route, have a duration of action of 2 weeks and should be preferred for preparation of patients to major surgery, or in the treatment of severe bleeding episodes because of their long-lasting effect.

10 BONE AND JOINT PROBLEMS

Bone involvement, historically called renal osteodystrophy, develops to some extent in all patients with end-stage renal failure and persists or even worsens during hemodialysis therapy. Uremia-related disorders of calcium, phosphate and vitamin D metabolism result in secondary hyperparathyroidism characterized by osteitis fibrosa, a high turnover bone disease. Aluminum overload, a frequent hazard during the seventies, inhibits mineralization of the bone matrix at the origin of osteomalacia. In some cases aluminum seems able to suppress parathyroid gland activity and a low turnover bone disease may ensue of such condition. Today, however, adynamic bone disease is increasingly observed in the absence of aluminum intoxication (Table 10–1). Another late, still incompletely elucidated complication is amyloid-related arthropathy.

TABLE 10-1. Main types of bone disease in dialysis patients

Type of disorder	Morphologic features	Etiopathogeny
Normal or high turnover		
mild	increased osteoid surface	vitamin D deficiency, mild hyperparathyroidism
osteitis fibrosa	bone marrow fibrosis	severe hyperparathyroidism
Low turnover		
aplastic (adynamic)	low bone formation rate	aluminum-induced, and/or depressed PTH secretion
osteomalacia	increased unmineralized osteoid	aluminum overload

Secondary hyperparathyroidism

Pathogenesis

The pathogenesis of hyperparathyroidism secondary to chronic renal failure is multifactorial.

> The two main consequences of reduced renal mass that contribute to the overfunctioning of the parathyroid glands are impaired phosphate elimination and decreased serum concentration of calcitriol (1,25(OH)2D3), the active metabolite of vitamin D.

Decreased calcitriol secretion, due to deficient 1a-hydroxylase activity of the diseased kidneys, leads to lower intestinal calcium absorption and decreased serum concentration of ionized calcium, thus stimulating PTH secretion. Moreover uremia is believed to be associated with a shift of the "set point" for calcium-mediated PTH secretion, a higher Ca++ level being required to suppress PTH release (Table 10–2). Additional factors involved in the development of hyperparathyroidism are relative resistance to the action of PTH on bone, a still controversed decrease of calcitriol receptors in the uremic parathyroid glands, and an hypothetical disturbance of the recently cloned calcium sensor receptor located on the parathyroid cell membrane (Figure 10–1).

Phosphate retention due to reduced active nephron mass inhibits calcitriol synthesis, therefore stimulating PTH secretion. In addition, hyperphosphatemia depresses serum calcium concentration and also possibly directly stimulates PTH secretion.

> Patients with advanced renal failure who have not been preventively treated with calcium and/or vitamin D supplements generally present with hypocalcemia, hyperphosphatemia and markedly increased serum PTH concentration.

TABLE 10-2. Causes and mechanisms of elevated PTH secretion in chronic renal failure

Stimuli	Pathogenic mechanism(s)
Hyperphosphatemia	Reduced phosphate excretion (nephron loss)
Hypocalcemia	Low calcitriol, hyperphosphatemia
Low serum calcitriol	Reduced renal mass, phosphate retention
Shift of the calcemic setpoint for PTH	Reduced sensitivity of calcium sensor receptors (uremic toxicity?)
Skeletal resistance to PTH	Low calcitriol, hyperphosphatemia, impaired PTH receptors (uremic toxicity?)
Reduced PTH degradation	Reduced renal mass

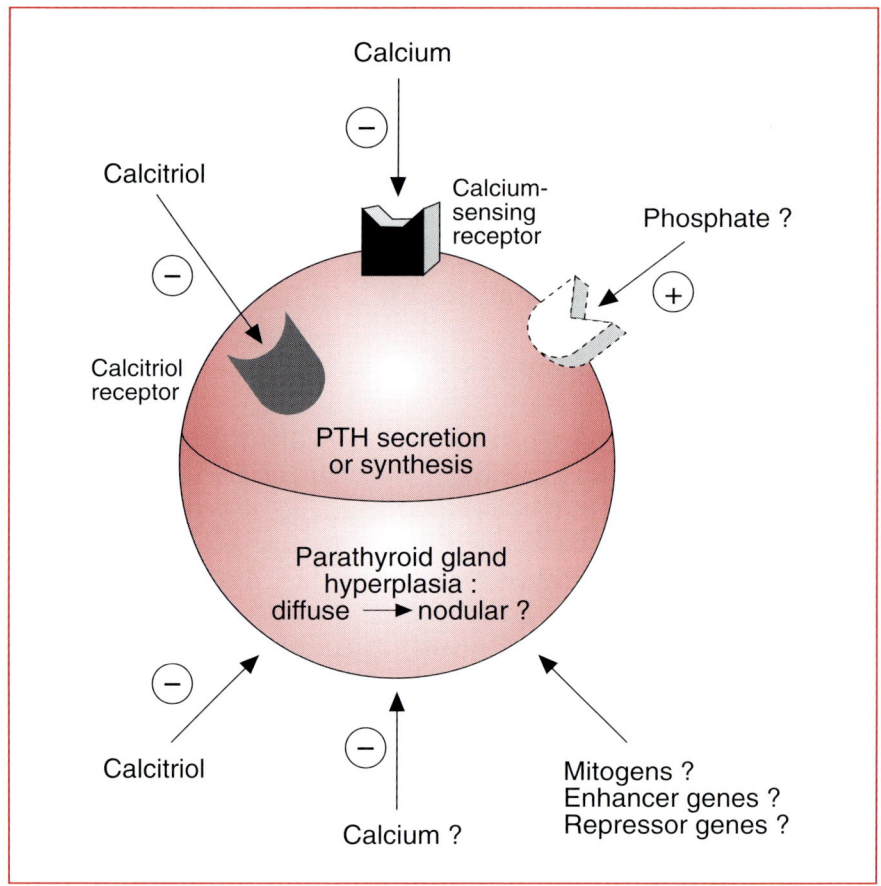

Figure 10-1: Regulation of parathyroid hormone (PTH) secretion. (+)=stimulation, (—)=inhibition. [Adapted from Drüeke T & Zingraff J. Current Opinion in Nephrology and Hypertension 3: 386–395, 1994, with permission].

Clinical presentation

Clinical and radiological signs occur only at very high PTH levels, more than ten times the upper limit of normal range (10–65 pg/ml for intact PTH). Clinical symptoms include bone pain (knees and heals are typically concerned), muscular weakness and itching, the latter attributed to skin deposits of calcium-phosphate crystals due to high serum phosphate concentration. Rupture of the tendon of the femoral quadriceps may occur in severe cases.

The most characteristic radiologic feature of osteitis fibrosa is sub-periosteal resorption of the cortex of digital phalanges, erosion of the external extremities of the claviculae and a mottled appearance of the skull. Painful periarticular calcifications may occur in patients with a high calcium phosphate product (> 70).

> Increased serum alkaline phosphatase, a marker of osteoblastic activity, indicates that hyperparathyroidism is a high turnover bone disease. The most reliable diagnostic criterion is the increase in serum concentration of intact parathyroid hormone (PTH 1–84), well correlated to cellular activity of bone so that usually bone biopsy is not required to establish the diagnosis.

Prophylactic treatment

Appropriate measures may prevent hyperparathyroidism if applied early, ideally before the start of dialysis (Table 10–3).

> Two goals are of primary importance. First, to maintain serum calcium at a sufficiently high level to suppress PTH overproduction, i.e., in the range of 2.4 to 2.7 mmol/l (9.6 to 10.8 mg/dl). Second, to control the serum phosphorus level by reducing intestinal absorption and promoting dialysis clearance, in order that serum phosphate should not exceed 1.8 mmol/l (5.6 mg/dl).

TABLE 10-3. Optimal calcium, phosphate and PTH serum levels for prevention of hyperparathyroidism

Calcium	2.4–2.7 mmol/l (9.6–10.8 mg/dl)
Phosphate	≤ 1.8 mmol/l (5.6 mg/dl)
Calcium-phosphorus product	< 70
Intact PTH	100–200 pg/ml (2–3 times the upper normal limit)
25 0H vit D3	>10 ng/ml

> Aluminum-containing phosphate binders should be avoided or administered only at low dose and for limited periods, in order to prevent the risk of aluminum intoxication.

Calcium salt supplements have the double beneficial effect of increasing serum calcium and decreasing phosphorus absorption, because calcium salts combine with phosphate anions in the intestinal lumen, thus acting as safe phosphate binders.

The most widely used calcium salt is calcium carbonate at a daily dose of 2 to 6 g, supplying 0.8 to 2.4 g elemental calcium per day. Calcium acetate may also be used at a lower dose. To maximize phosphate binding, calcium supplements should be given with animal protein-containing meals. In addition a prudent dose of calcitriol or of alfacalcidol (0.25 or 0.50 µg/day) may help to maintain serum PTH level in the optimal range of 100 to 200 pg/ml.

Such measures usually suffice to maintain serum calcium, phosphorus and PTH at the targeted level. However, when not timely applied, overt secondary hyperparathyroidism may develop thus requiring specific therapeutic measures.

Treatment of overt secondary hyperparathyroidism

> As long as serum calcium and phosphorus concentrations are not elevated beyond any control, medical treatment is indicated.

High dose calcium supplements should be used, together with calcitriol or alfacalcidol supplied either daily, or as pulse therapy at the end of dialysis sessions. The superiority of the intravenous over the oral route has as yet not been established. Anyhow, the effect of calcium and vitamin D supplementation should be rigorously monitored in order to avoid excessive calcium and phosphate serum concentrations.

> When high dose $CaCO_3$ supplements are used, dialysate calcium concentration should be lowered e.g., to 1.25 mmol/l (50 mg/l) in order to limit the total calcium uptake. However, such low calcium dialysates should be used only in compliant patients, able to ingest the required dose of oral calcium supplements, otherwise a negative calcium balance may ensue.

When drug therapy fails to control PTH level or does so at the unacceptable price of excessive hypercalcemia and/or hyperphosphatemia, reduction of parathyroid glands is indicated, the more so if the patient has developed diffuse extraskeletal (especially vascular) calcifications, severe skeletal or muscular pain and/or intractable pruritus. Subtotal parathyroidectomy is the most employed strategy but some groups prefer total parathyroidectomy associated or not with forearm autotransplantation of parathyroid fragments. Recently, successful reduction of hyperparathyroidism by alcohol instillation in enlarged glands under ultrasonic guidance has been reported.

Aluminum-related osteomalacia

Since the widespread use of active vitamin D analogs in uremic patients, vitamin D deficient osteomalacia characterized by increased osteoid, poor matrix mineralization and increased PTH has virtually disappeared.

Aluminum (Al) intoxication is now the most frequent cause of osteomalacia in dialysis patients. The deleterious effects of aluminum poisoning add to, and interfere with secondary hyperparathyroidism. The main causes of Al intoxication are summarized in Table 10-4.

TABLE 10-4. Causes of aluminum intoxication

Aluminum-contaminated dialysis fluid
Aluminum-containing phosphate binders
Concomitant ingestion of calcium citrate (or orther citrate salts) and aluminum- containing drugs as antacids or phosphate binders

Pathophysiology and diagnosis

Bone biopsy with double labeling (two doses of tetracycline two weeks apart prior to biopsy) shows a marked excess of unmineralized osteoid. Al is located as a band at the limit of osteoid and calcified tissue, inhibiting normal mineralization. Low plasma concentrations of PTH and alcaline phosphatases designate this Al related, vitamin D-resistant osteomalacia as a low-turnover bone disease.

Of note, Al poisoning reduces the degree of hyperparathyroidism by reducing PTH release. On the other hand, hyperparathyroidism attenuates bone toxicity of Al so that worsening of Al bone disease is often seen after parathyroidectomy.

Al intoxication is associated with severe bone and joint pain. Fractures of the ribs are frequent. Microcytic anemia and encephalopathy may coexist.

Diagnosis of Al overload is based on deferoxamine (DFO) test, serum Al concentrations being only indicative. Although serum Al concentrations over 60 µg/l (normal value < 10 µg/l) are usually associated with Al accumulation, there is no tight correlation between Al serum level and degree of Al accumulation.

After infusion of 5 mg/kg of deferoxamine in isotonic glucose over 60 min, an increment in serum Al (measured at the start of the next hemodialysis session) over 150 µg/l is indicative of significantly increased tissue Al stores.

Treatment of aluminum accumulation

> The best treatment is prophylactic by avoidance, or strict limitation of all Al-containing phosphate binders or antacid drugs, and use of deionized water containing less than 8 µg/l (0.3 µmol/l) of Al.

Al accumulation documented by the DFO test should be treated by discontinuation of any Al source and regular DFO therapy, by means of 5–10 mg/kg BW of DFO in isotonic glucose infused during the last 60 min of a dialysis session once a week.

Serum Al concentration must be regularly checked during DFO therapy and kept below 400 µg/l (15 µmol/l) to avoid the risk of exacerbating or precipitating Al-related encephalopathy. Prolonged therapy may increase susceptibility to Yersinia sepsis and mucormycosis, because DFO interfers with iron metabolism. Attention should be paid also to the possible retinal and auditory toxicity of the drug.

Adynamic bone disease

An aplastic form of osteodystrophy is increasingly reported during the last years. Such adynamic bone disease is characterized by the virtual absence of osteoblastic and osteoclastic cell activity, with low bone formation and lack of increase in osteoid volume. This lesion is mainly a histologic finding, and usually asymptomatic. Although the precise pathogenesis of the disorder still remains to be elucidated, depressed PTH concentration seems to be a prerequisite for the development of aplastic bone. Initially thought to result from Al intoxication, a possible explanation was found in the suppressive effect of Al on parathyroid gland function. However, in most cases such adynamic bone disease occurs today independently of any Al overload, probably reflecting an excessive correction of hyperparathyroidism by calcitriol and/or CaCO3 therapy. Diabetes mellitus and peritoneal dialysis are additional risk factors.

Beta 2-microglobulin amyloidosis

The incidence of dialysis-related beta 2-microglobulin (β2-m) amyloidosis in patients with end-stage renal failure maintained on long-term hemodialysis is steadily increasing during the past ten years.

Clinical manifestations

Clinical signs and symptoms concern mainly articular and juxta-articular structures. Carpal tunnel syndrome (CTS), the most common manifestation, is revealed by paresthesias, pain and numbness in the hands. Exacerbation during night or during dialysis sessions is characteristic. Median nerve conduction velocity is diagnostic. Surgical release of the median nerve is the treatment of choice. Tenosynovitis of finger flexors may develop and results in "trigger fingers".

Arthropathy involves large joints such as shoulders, knees, elbows and hips, but also wrists, often concomitant to CTS. Erosive cysts are frequent in humeral heads, acetabulum, femoral head and neck, carpal bones, and may result in pathologic fractures.

Spondylarthropathy, mainly affecting the cervical spine, is found to be often associated to β2-m amyloid deposits. Computed tomography and magnetic resonance imaging are more useful to demonstrate the extent of the lesions than plain X-rays. Ultrasonic echography allows early detection of synovial thickening due to amyloid infiltration especially of the shoulder and hip joints.

Pathogenesis and risk factors

The major fibrillar constituent protein of this unique type of amyloid has been identified as β2-m. The sole known route to clear the β2-m molecule is via the kidneys, hence in advanced renal failure β2-m accumulates as an ongoing function of time. Plasma concentration reaches very high values, particularly in anurics, up to more than 30 fold the upper limit of the normal range (1 to 2 mg/l). Risk factors for β2-m amyloidosis are summarized in Table 10-5.

TABLE 10-5. Risk factors for β2-m amyloidosis

Retention of β2-m (poor dialysis extraction)

Older age of the patient

Increased duration on hemodialysis

Stimulation of inflammatory mediators (cytokines, proteases and reactive oxygen species) by complement-activating membranes and/or bacterial endotoxins

Iron or aluminum overload

Hyperparathyroidism

> Low-flux cellulosic membranes do not allow extraction of b2-m. Futhermore these bioincompatible membranes via complement activation and phagocyte release of proteases and reactive oxygen species may enhance b2-m production and amyloid fibril formation. By contrast, high-flux, biocompatible membranes such as polyacrylonitrile (AN69), polysulfone or PMMA allow partial extraction of b2-m and probably do not trigger b2-m generation.

Kidney transplantation restores renal catabolism of β2-m and is associated with relief of joint pain. However, inspite of almost normal serum β2-m levels abundant amyloid tissue deposits can be found in synovial structures more than ten years after transplantation. Although β2-m retention is obviously a prerequisite for the development of β2-m amyloidosis, factors determining the elective predilection of β2-m amyloid for joints and adjacent bone (at variance with all other types of amyloidosis) are still poorly understood. Of note β2-M amyloidosis has been occasionally observed before any renal replacement therapy in patients with longstanding renal failure.

> Patient's age at the start of dialysis and duration of dialysis treatment are major determinants for the development b2-m amyloidosis which is virtually constant beyond 15 years on hemodialysis. However, several groups have reported a lower incidence of b2-m amyloidosis, at comparable dialysis duration, when using biocompatible membranes (Figure 10–2).

The use of biocompatible, highly permeable membranes is recommended in all patients at risk for developing β2-m amyloidosis, such as those who are not waiting for a kidney graft, and even more so for patients who already have evidence of the disease.

Other osteoarticular problems

Soft tissue calcifications

Three types of soft tissue calcification can be distinguished: vascular calcifications (mainly of median sized arteries), visceral calcifications affecting heart, lung and kidney, and periarticular calcifications that may grow to pseudotumoral size. Although factors leading to such calcium deposits are poorly known, hyperphosphatemia plays a pathogenic role. Individual susceptibility to develop ectopic calcifications differs from one

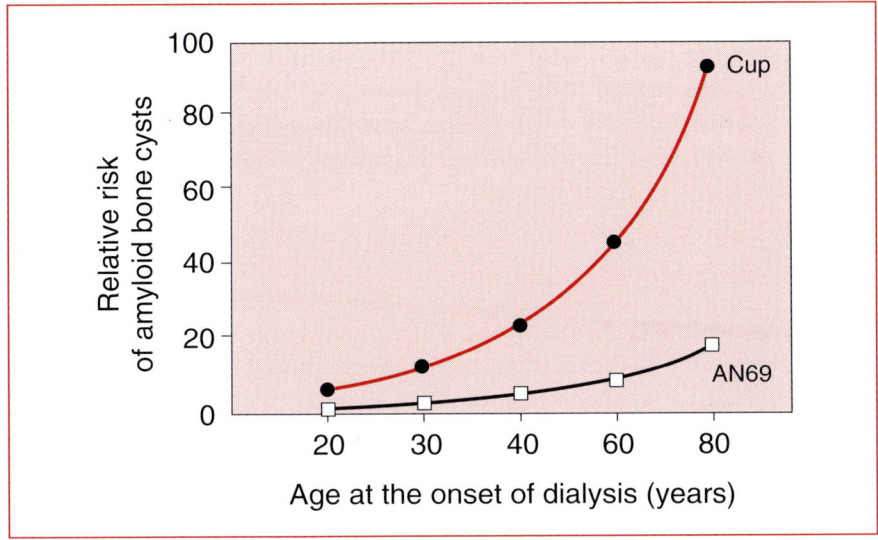

Figure 10-2: Relative risk of developing radiological signs of bone amyloidosis as a function of age at the initiation of dialysis either on AN69 or on Cuprophane(Cup) membrane. [Adapted from Van Ypersele de Strihou C et al. Kidney Int 39: 1012–1019, 1991, with permission].

patient to the other. Historically attributed to uncontrolled hyperparathyroidism, extraskeletal calcifications are now more frequently observed in the absence of PTH excess and more likely result from inhibited calcium uptake by the skeleton as is the case in adynamic bone disease.

Phosphate is not the only anion able to form crystals leading to inflammatory lesions. Oxalate and urate serum concentrations are also increased in dialysis patients and precipitation of oxalate and urate crystals may induce microcrystalline arthropathy.

Secondary gout

Uric acid accumulation may result in uric acid deposits in joints and gouty attacks. Allopurinol can be used to lower serum acid concentration because its main metabolite, oxypurinol, is readily extracted by hemodialysis and therefore the risk of cutaneous untoward effects is much lower than in predialysis uremic patients.

Osteoporosis and bone fluorosis

When cumulated to the hereabove mentioned lesions osteoporosis may worsen bone fragility of long-term dialysis patients. Osteoporosis may be steroid-related in patients who experienced graft rejection, or age-related, especially in the elderly woman in whom substitutive hormonal therapy should be recommended to limit bone loss.

Bone fluorosis is a rare complication which may result from an excessive drinking of fluorid-rich water during the period of advanced renal failure prior to dialysis.

Destructive spondylarthropathy

Destructive spondylarthropathy is a frequent lesion typical for mixed osteo-arthropathy, with elements of osteitis fibrosa, amyloidosis and osteoporosis in variable combination. Severe cases, with neurological signs of medullar or radicular compression, require surgical consolidation by an interbody fusion procedure using autologous iliac bone grafts.

> A close cooperation between nephrologists, rheumatologists and orthopedic surgeons is required for the optimal management of such multiple, often invalidating osteoarticular problems.

11 OTHER CLINICAL PROBLEMS

Endocrine disorders

Circulating levels of total T4 and T3 are usually low, but free T4 and T3 concentrations are normal, as are reverse T3 and TSH basal levels. Significant hypothyroidism is not a frequent event in uremic patients.

By contrast, pituitary-gonadal axis is markedly impaired in both male and female ESRD patients. Male patients frequently have low plasma testosterone levels, and complain of reduced libido and impotence. Erectile dysfunction may also result from cavernous occlusive arterial disease as evidenced by angiography.

Female patients are now rarely amenorrheic, but often have functional menorrhagias which contribute to anemia. Intermittent or continuous prescription of progestogens compensates for luteal insufficiency and prevents unwanted blood loss. In both sexes, hyperprolactinemia is reported in a variable percentage of cases, sometimes associated to gynecomastia or galactorrhea. Anemia contributes to impaired sexual activity as shown by the improvement usually following r-HuEPO therapy.

Due to improved fertility, pregnancy is now less exceptional than in the past in chronic dialysis female patients. Spontaneous abortion is still a frequent issue. However a successful outcome is presently obtained in an increasing number of cases, thanks to a close cooperation between nephrologists, obstetricians and neonatologists. Conditions that contribute to an improved outcome of pregnancy are listed in Table 11–1.

TABLE 11-1. Conditions to optimize pregnancy outcome in a dialysis patient

Maintain blood urea under 20 mmol/l by frequent dialysis to prevent polyhydramnios
Use no or prudent heparinization
Increase protein and calorie supply
Correct anemia (iron and folate supplements, r-HuEPO)
Adapt antihypertensive medication (avoid ACEI)

Metabolic disorders

Carbohydrate metabolism is impaired in ESRD, with glucose intolerance and insulin resistance at the post-receptor level, due to uremic toxins. Hyperinsulinism may contribute to atherogenesis.

Altered lipid metabolism is a major risk factor for atherogenesis, because hypertriglyceridemia concomitant to altered lipoprotein pattern (with decreased apoAI and AII and increased apoB, CII, CIII and E levels) is considered to be atherogenic and manifests from the early stage of renal failure. Reduced intake of rapidly absorbed carbohydrates, preferred use of unsaturated fats (such as olive or colza oils) and polyunsaturated fats (including fish oil) instead of saturated fats is indicated. In the case of marked hypertriglyceridemia and/or hypercholesterolemia, prudent therapy with respectively fibrates or HMGCo reductase inhibitors may be required; dosage should be reduced accordingly to decreased excretion.

Hyperhomocysteinemia, which is constantly present in uremics and is only partially reduced by hemodialysis, acts as an independent atherogenic factor. Pharmacologic supplementation with folic acid (2-5 mg/day) substantially lowers plasma homocysteine concentration and should be of interest independent of hematologic indications.

> Incompletely compensated chronic metabolic acidosis is frequent in dialysis patients. Acidosis enhances protein catabolism, especially in skeletal muscle, and thus contributes to negative nitrogen balance and malnutrition.

Dermatological problems

Uremic pruritus

Pruritus is frequent in dialysis patients. Its origin is multifactorial. The most commonly advocated mechanism is deposition of calcium-phosphate crystals in the skin, in the context of overt secondary hyperparathyroidism with marked hyperphosphatemia. Other contributing mechanisms are listed in Table 11–2. If adequate control of hyperphosphatemia is ineffective to relieve pruritus, one should prescribe topical emollients to cure skin dryness, evict identified allergens, change heparin specialty, or use oral antipruritic drugs.

TABLE 11-2. Etiology of uremic pruritus

Deposition of calcium-phosphate crystals in the skin (hyperparathyroidism, hyperphosphatemia)
Dryness of the skin
Drug allergy (heparin, ethylene oxide)
Histamine release from mast cells

Bullous dermatoses

Uremic pseudoporphyria is an acquired, uremia-related form of porphyria cutanea tarda manifested by vesicles and bullae developed on sunlight-exposed part of the skin, which may progress to severe ulcerating lesions. Iron overload is a major pathogenic factor, because an iron-dependent oxidative mechanism inactivates the hepatic enzyme uroporphyrinogen-decarboxylase, thus resulting in increased levels of plasma porphyrins (with their high photosensitivity potential) due to the lack of urine excretion and poor dialysis extraction (Figure 11–1). Treatment relies on combined phlebotomy and r-HuEPO, which allows to deplete liver iron stores more rapidly than DFO therapy.

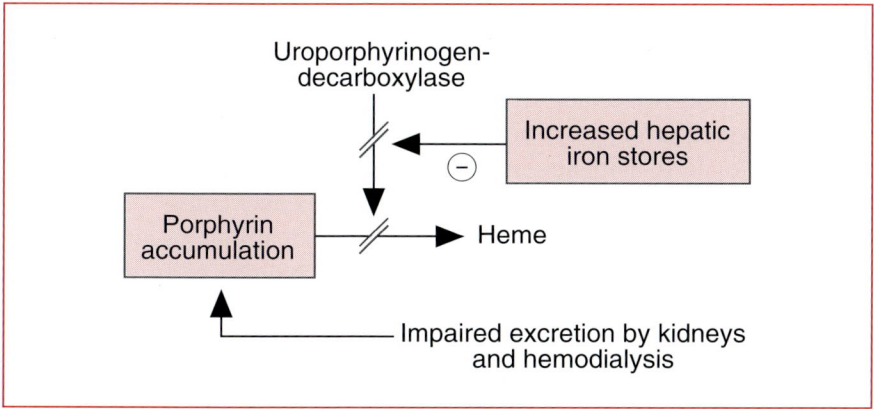

Figure 11-1: Mechanism of porphyrin accumulation in hemodialysis patients with liver iron overload.

Gastrointestinal complications

Functional disorders

GI symptoms are frequent at the advanced stage of renal failure, mainly in the form of anorexia, morning nausea, vomiting and altered taste (dysgueusia), all of which may lead to malnutrition. A metallic taste in the mouth sometimes leads to inappropriate polydipsia and excessive water intake. Dyspepsia is frequent, with post-prandial eructations, pyrosis and regurgitation, due to underlying oesophagitis, hiatal hernia and/or gastritis. Gastric acid secretion is increased in dialysis patients, mainly due to decreased levels of gastric inhibitory peptide (an inhibitor of acid secretion which is removed by hemodialysis), whereas gastrin secretion itself is increased.

> Constipation is a frequent problem, especially in older patients, favored by ingestion of large quantities of phosphate-binder powders, reduction in vegetable and fruit intake to avoid hyperkalemia, and sedentarity.

Peptic ulcer disease is more frequent in ESRD patients than in the general population but usually responds well to antacid therapy and H_2-receptor antagonists. Of note, antacids interfer with iron absorption, and omeprazole therapy causes malabsorption of vitamin B12.

> Upper GI tract endoscopy is indicated in every patient with persistent dyspeptic symptoms, and prior to kidney transplantation.

GI bleeding

A major probem is bleeding from the GI tract. The causes are the same as for dyspeptic disorders. In addition, some causes should be especially sought in dialysis patients, namely telangectasias and angiodysplasia, which can only be shown by endoscopy; ischemic colitis (favored by atherosclerosis and/or β2m amyloidosis); pseudomembranous colitis due to clostridium difficile; stercoral ulcers with colonic perforation, and diverticulitis.

> Diverticulitis is especially frequent in patients with polycystic kidney disease and differential diagnosis with kidney cyst infection may be difficult.

> Endoscopy is the key investigation to identify the location and cause of upper as well as lower GI tract bleeding.

Other digestive complications

Chronic pancreatitis is frequent in ESRD patients, and acute pancreatitis occurs in about 2% of them. Because basal serum amylase level is often elevated in ESRD patients, lipase which is less influenced by renal failure should be of more help for diagnosis. Besides chronic virus C, virus B and/or CMV hepatitis, drug-induced liver alteration is frequent. Silicone particles from blood pumps may accumulate in the liver and provoke hepatic granulomatosis. Hepatic cysts may provoke septic complications and/or compression of intra or extrahepatic biliary ducts or inferior vena cava. Differential diagnosis with complications of polycystic kidneys is difficult and may be helped by CT scan and/or magnetic resonance imaging.

Complications in the diseased kidneys

Acquired cystic kidney disease

Development of multiple acquired cysts in previously non-cystic kidneys is a common long-term complication of ESRD of any etiology. The number and size of acquired cysts increase with time on dialysis. Pathogenesis involves compensatory hypertrophy of residual nephrons and proximal tubule epithelial cell hyperplasia mediated by increased production of, or increased sensitivity to, local growth factors. In addition, tubular obstruction by albumin and/or $\beta2$-microglobulin concretions may play a role. Such hyperplasia may be a precursor to the development of renal tumors. Bleeding (including retroperitoneal hematoma) and renal cell carcinoma are the most deleterious clinical complications (Table 11–3). Thus, echography and CT scan are needed for all dialysis patients with unexplained hematuria, abdominal pain or blood loss.

TABLE 11-3. Complications of acquired kidney cysts

Bleeding (mild hematuria up to perirenal hematoma)
Erythrocytosis (especially post-transplantation)
Renal cell carcinoma (male predominance)

> Ideally, abdominal echography and CT scan should be obtained at start of dialysis as reference, and repeated every 3 years, or sooner in case of hematuria or unexplained lumbar pain.

Kidney stones

Formation of kidney stones, usually made of a mixture of calcium oxalate and matrix proteins, is not infrequent in ESRD patients, but is rarely of clinical consequence because small proteinaceous stones are easily passed. The main risk factors for the development of such stones are high protein concentration and/or increased calcium concentration in residual urine due to vit D3 therapy, in the face of the unavoidable high urinary oxalate concentration due to hyperoxalemia.

Psychological problems

Facing the need for indefinitely sustained dialysis is always a distressing and frustating situation. Anxiety is almost always present in hemodialysis patients. The feeling of body integrity is altered by the vascular access and connexion to the dialysis machine. Loss of urine emission is sorely experienced especially by men. A depressive tendency is often associated. Depression can be expressed as aggressivity toward the medical staff or relatives, or as opposition in diet and treatment.Depression may also be a reaction to social, familial and/or professionnal problems, aggravated by the constraints arising from dialysis.

> Regular conversation with the patient to allow him to express his fears, and psychological support are essential for the success of treatment.The aid of social workers to recover a job or solving social problems is of primary interest.

It must be stressed that depressive manifestations per se should not justify withdrawal of therapy. However the decision to discontinue dialysis may be considered in patients with severe and irreversible deterioration of physical and mental condition as can been seen in very aged subjects.

Dialysis in children

Maintenance hemodialysis can be used in the child as an alternative to peritoneal dialysis. Specific problems have to be overcome.

Technical problems

Blood access is often a difficult problem. Dual-lumen internal jugular vein catheter is now the most common permanent access used in younger children. Pediatric hemodialyzers must have a small blood volume and the blood content of the entire extracorporal circuit should not exceed 10–15% of the total blood volume of the child. Low blood flow rate should be used, according to child's body size and strict control of ultrafiltration rate is mandatory. Psychologic support during dialysis sessions is needed in young children.

Metabolic problems

Protein and calorie supply requirements are comparatively higher than in adults, with an optimal protein intake of 2 g/kg BW/day. Vitamin D supplementation and correction of acidosis are essential for growth. In addition, bioavailability of growth hormone in ESRD children is impaired, due to reduced production and/or presence of uremic toxins acting as inhibitors of somatomedin activity. Therefore, statural growth of uremic children may be markedly impaired, especially when severe failure is present at the prepubertal age.

> Fortunately, recombinant human growth hormone (r-HuGH) now allows to dramatically improve growth rate in uremic children (Figure 11-2). Of note, treatment should be initiated early in the predialysis stage as soon as GFR is less than 30 ml/min/1.73m^2. Improvement in growth velocity persists after initiation of dialysis. Combined with the use of r-HuEPO when needed, r-HuGH therapy is one of the most significant advances in the management of pediatric uremic patients in the past few years.

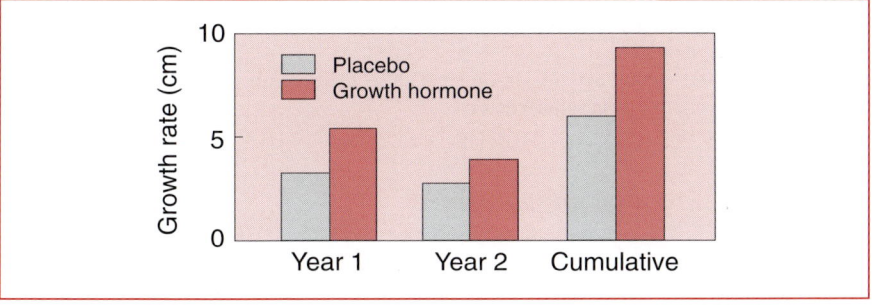

Figure 11-2: Effects of recombinant growth hormone on height in ESRD children. [Data provided by Genentech Inc, San Francisco, CA].

Dialysis in the elderly

Obviously, the number of elderly patients accepted on dialysis programs is constantly growing, as their proportion in the general population grows in industrialized countries. At the present time, more than half of the patients starting maintenance dialysis are aged 60 years or more. Moreover, the incidence of ESRD markedly rises with age. The overall rate is about 150 per million under 50 years of age, and greater than 500 per million in subjects over 65.

> The increase is the most marked in the oldest age class, i.e., patients aged 75 years or more, who are the most exposed to multiple co-morbid conditions and dialysis-associated complications.

There are essentially no specific problems due to age, because the physiological and psychological status of the individual patient is largely independent of age. A number of patients over 65 are able to be treated by home dialysis or limited-care dialysis, and to benefit from kidney transplantation. Most problems arise in very old patients with limited autonomy, especially when no familial support exists. Some general precautions may help to improve tolerance and benefits of treatment in the aged population (Table 11–4).

TABLE 11-4. Strategies to optimize maintenance hemodialysis in elderly subjects

Use bicarbonate-buffered dialysate
Use high dialysate sodium concentration ($\geq$ 142 mEq/l)
Closely monitor blood pressure during dialysis sessions
Avoid rapid ultrafiltration (avoid excessive interdialytic weight gain)
Avoid post prandial hypotension
Treat anemia (Hb level no less than 9 g/dl)
Provide adequate protein-calorie nutrition (intradialytic aminoacid supplementation if needed)
Provide vitamin supplements (including vit B12, vit B6 and folates)
Identify and treat depression
Sustain physical and mental activity (in-center dialysis helps compensate for loneliness)
Avoid polypharmacy and drug interferences

Dialysis in the diabetic patient

Growing incidence of diabetic ESRF

Patients with diabetic nephropathy constitute the most rapidly growing fraction of ESRD patients beginning dialysis therapy in the recent years, at least in the United States and Northern European countries. As an example, the proportion of diabetics within the total number of ESRD patients in the USA has grown from 20.5% in 1987 to 24.5% in 1990 and 34.3% in 1993. Diabetic nephropathy is now the leading cause of ESRD in the USA. The incidence of diabetic nephropathy is 3 to 7 times higher in Blacks than in Whites.

> Diabetes adds its own complications to those of chronic uremia, namely polyneuritis, retinopathy, and coronary, cerebrovascular and peripheral macroangiopathy. Coronary artery and cerebrovascular disease is responsible for more than half of the mortality observed in dialyzed diabetics.

Management of the diabetic dialysis patient

Due to the accelerated progression of retinopathy and neuropathy in diabetics with advanced renal failure, dialysis should be initiated earlier than in other uremics, ideally when serum creatinine concentration reaches 500–700 µmol/l ($\approx$ 5.5 to 8 mg/dl). Accordingly, vascular access should be created long in advance.

Insulin delivery must be adjusted to individual requirements. Typically, ESRD diabetic patients experience decreased renal catabolism of insulin and dialysis improves tissue insulin sensitivity, thus resulting in decreased insulin need. However, improved appetite may be a counterbalance and result in increased insulin requirement. Optimal glycemic control is needed in diabetic patients on dialysis in order to minimize thirst (and consequent excessive interdialytic weight gain), avoid ketoacidosis, and limit lipid metabolism disturbances. In assessing the quality of glycemic control, the measurement of glycosylated hemoglobin (hemoglobin A1C) may be confused by retention of carbamylated hemoglobins, whereas fructosamine, another indicator of glycemic control, is less affected by renal failure.

> A multidisciplinary approach involving close cooperation between nephrologist, diabetologist, dietician, ophtalmologist, cardiologist, podiatrist and vascular surgeon is needed to improve survival and quality of life of the diabetic patient on long-term dialysis.

12 OUTCOME AND ECONOMICS

Long survival and optimal quality of life afforded to the dialysis patient are the main concerns in maintenance hemodialysis.

Results of maintenance hemodialysis

Survival of patients on hemodialysis

> There is no theoretical limitation to the length of survival of patients on maintenance hemodialysis. Ideally, the combined effects of improved technology and intensive medical surveillance should allow to overcome uremia-induced complications and to approach the life expectancy of subjects of similar age devoided of renal disease.

As a matter of fact, several thousands of dialysis patients have survived more than 10 years, and hundreds more than 20 years. Several of our patients are still living over 25 years on hemodialysis, and enjoy life.

The overall annual mortality rate is about 5% in European and Japanese patients and appears to be stable over years, because the increasing proportion of older patients counterbalances the positive effects of improved technology. As expected, mortality rate increases with age, as shown on Figure 12–1 illustrating survival of dialysis patients of various age in our dialysis unit and associate facilities in the recent past years. Comorbid conditions also adversely affect survival.

The annual mortality rate is reported to be much higher in the United States, with a mean value close to 20%. This difference with European reports cannot entirely be explained by a higher proportion of elderly and

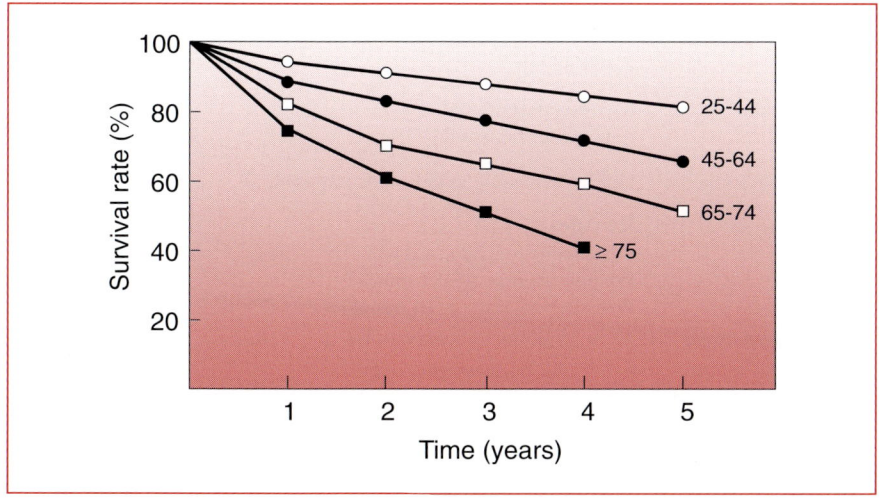

Figure 12-1: Actuarial survival of patients according to age at start of hemodialysis (Necker Hospital and associate centers, patients started on dialysis between 1986–1989).

diabetic patients, as it persists after adjustement on all variables. A plausible explanation is that a number of patients in the USA do not receive truly adequate dialysis due to a weekly dialysis time lower than in Europe or Japan (9 hours as a mean vs 12 to 15 hours). Recent prospective studies in the USA clearly show that an effective duration of dialysis sessions of no less than 4 hours with a Kt/V of at least 1.2 was associated with a dramatic improvement in survival, with annual mortality rate decreasing from 22.8% to 9.1% over 3 years.

A consensus emerges that excessive shortening of the duration of dialysis sessions, to 3 hours or less, does not allow sufficient clearance of uremic toxins, especially those which behave as "middle molecules", even if Kt/V urea (or URR) seems to be adequate, because such kinetic analysis is only based on the extraction of a rapidly cleared molecule.

Conditions that should ideally provide the best survival to dialysis patients are summarized in Table 12–1.

Quality of life and rehabilitation

The quality of life of dialysis patients has substantially improved with time, due to higher efficiency of dialyzers, use of bicarbonate buffer, better

TABLE 12-1. Conditions for optimal hemodialysis

Blood flow	: ≥ 300 ml/min
Dialysis fluid	: bicarbonate-buffered non-pyrogenic, sterile
Dialysis membrane	: highly permeable, highly biocompatible
Dose of dialysis	: Kt/Vurea: ≥ 1.2 Urea reduction rate: ≥ 0.65 Predialysis urea: 30–35 mmol/l Post dialysis urea: 5–10 mmol/l
Weekly dialysis time	: 12 to 15 hours (3 sessions of 4 to 5 hours)
Daily protein intake	: ≥ 1.2 g/kg body weight

control of ultrafiltration, adjustment of sodium, more efficient blood pressure control, recombinant erythropoietin therapy and more attention given to the nutritional state with more reliable indicators.

As a consequence, most patients can resume full- or part-time activity, especially those treated by home dialysis who benefit from greater autonomy.

> Resuming or maintaining normal professional activity is not only an economic necessity for most dialysis patients, but is psychologically important. Therefore, all efforts should tend to facilitate social and familial rehabilitation.

Economics of dialysis therapy

Maintenance hemodialysis is today the most expensive of all medical treatments. Due to the continuously increasing number of new patients accepted on dialysis therapy, the cost of health care is in all countries mounting steadily.

Increasing needs of dialysis therapy

> The main factor is the continuously growing number of elderly patients accepted on dialysis programs, due to the generalized ageing of population in industrialized countries.

As an example, whereas subjects over 60 years of age represent only 25% of the population in France, they account for 54% of ESRD patients requiring supportive therapy (Figure 12–2).

The number of patients on dialysis therapy in the United States was

OUTCOME AND ECONOMICS

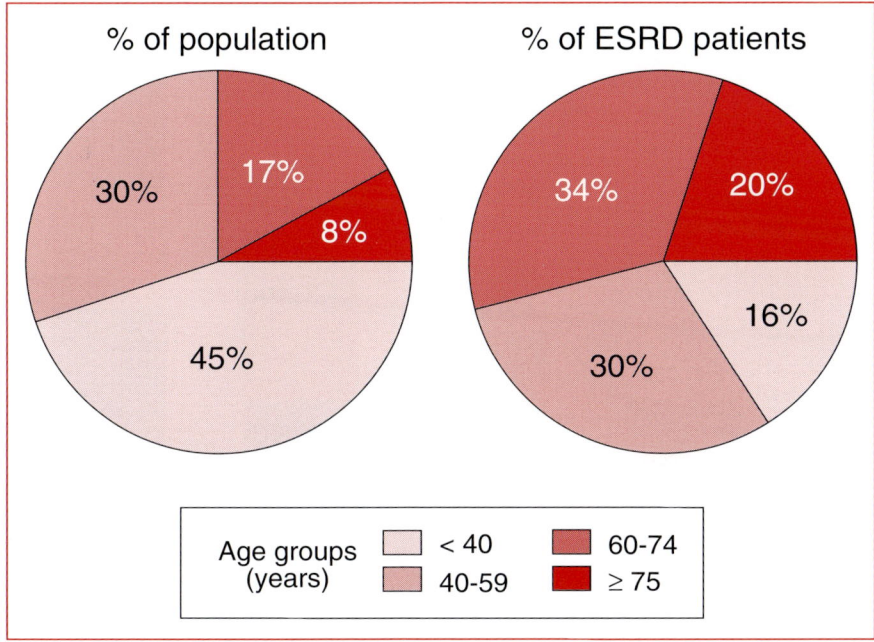

Figure 12-2: Relative incidence of ESRD with respect to age groups in the Paris area, France, 1992–1993.

about 10,000 in 1972, 96,000 in 1983 and 174,000 in 1993, for a total population of 249 millions. The annual growth rate was nearly 10% from 1980 to 1990, and the same increment is predicted from 1990 to 2000.

By the end of 1993, the total number of patients treated by dialysis worldwide was 590,000, including 505,000 on hemodialysis and 85,000 on peritoneal dialysis. North America, Japan and Europe accounted for more than three quarters of this total.

Figure 12–3 depicts the predictable progression of the number of patients treated worldwide by maintenance hemodialysis based on an average annual increment rate of 4% in Europe, 8% in Japan, 10% in the USA and 8% in other countries. Because the number of kidney transplantations performed does not progress at a similar rate, and because improved adequacy of dialysis partially abates the adverse effects of age and comorbidity on survival, the total number of dialysis-treated patients will possibly exceed 1 million worldwide at the end of this century.

The cost of dialysis therapy

The cost of dialysis therapy is considerable and constantly growing. Among the total number of patients treated all over the world by

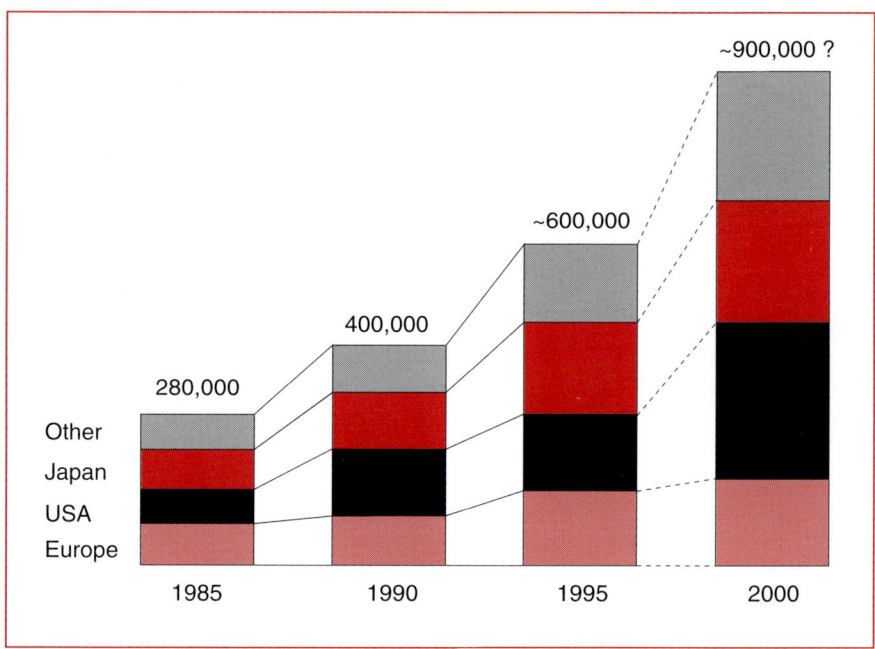

Figure 12-3: Projection of the overall prevalence of patients to be treated by maintenance hemodialysis at entry into the third millenium.

maintenance hemodialysis in 1993, about 80% were "in-center" treated. The total cost in the United States for 1993 was estimated to be near 6.5 billion dollars. On the basis of a similar cost in other countries, the total expense throughout the world may be estimated at 25 billion dollars at the same time, and may be expected to exceed 50 billion dollars at the beginning of the third millenium.

> These economic considerations do not in any way put in question the legitimacy of dialysis therapy and the right of the renal patient to be treated. However, they should make the public, doctors and industrial companies aware of such high cost and stimulate finding ways to lower the cost of the method while improving its efficacy, and to develop kidney transplantation.

In the future, intensive research efforts should be oriented to identify etiopathogenic factors of renal diseases in order to prevent such diseases and to arrest, or at least slow their progression to end-stage renal failure, thus decreasing the number of patients requiring supportive therapy.

LITERATURE FOR FURTHER READING

Recommended books for further reading:
Replacement of Renal Function by Dialysis, Jacobs C, Kjellstrand CM, Koch KM, Winchester JF (eds), Kluwer Academic Publishers, Dordrecht, The Netherlands, 4th edition, 1995.
Principles and Practice of Dialysis, Henrich WL (ed), Baltimore, Williams & Wilkins, 1994.

Chapters and articles
Abuelo JG, Shemin D, Chazan JA. Acute symptoms produced by hemodialysis: A review of their causes and associations. Semin Dial 6: 59–69, 1993.
Acchiardo SR, Moore LW, Latour PA. Malnutrition as the main factor in morbidity and mortality of hemodialysis patients. Kidney Int 24 (suppl 16): S199–S203, 1983.
Acchiardo SR. Uremia and adequate dialysis treatment. Semin Nephrol 14: 274–281, 1994.
Akmal M, Sawelson S, Karubian F, Gadallah M. The prevalence and significance of occult blood loss in patients with predialysis advanced chronic renal failure, or receiving dialysis therapy. Clin Nephrol 42: 198–202, 1994.
Anderson K, Goeger DE, Carson RW, Lee SK, Stead RB. Erythropoietin for the treatment of porphyria cutanea tarda in a patient on long-term hemodialysis. N Engl J Med 322: 315–317, 1990.
Avram MR, Pena C, Burrell D, Antignassi A, Avram MM. Hemodialysis in the elderly patient: Potential advantages as to quality of life, urea generation, serum creatinine and less interdialytic weight gain. Am J Kidney Dis 16: 342–345, 1990.
Babb AL, Ahmad S, Bergström J, Scribner BH. The middle molecular hypothesis in perspective. Am J Kidney Dis 1: 46–50, 1981.
Bander SJ, Schwab SJ. Central venous angioaccess for hemodialysis and its complications. Semin Dial 5: 121–128, 1992.
Bardin T, Zingraff J, Shirahama T, et al. Hemodialysis-associated amyloidosis and beta-2 microglobulin. Clinical and immuno-histochemical study. Am J Med 83: 419–424, 1987.

Basile C, Casino F, Lopez T. Percent reduction in blood urea concentration during dialysis estimates Kt/V in a simple and accurate way. Am J Kidney Dis 15: 40–45, 1990.

Bergström J, Alverstrand A, Fürst P. Plasma and muscle free amino acids in maintenance hemodialysis patients without protein malnutrition. Kidney Int 38: 108–114, 1990.

Brescia MJ, Cimino JE, Appel K, Hurwich BJ. Chronic hemodialysis using venipuncture and a surgically created arteriovenous fistula. N Engl J Med 275: 1089–1092, 1966.

Brown JH, Hunt LP, Vites NP, Short CD, Gokal R, Mallick NP. Comparative mortality from cardiovascular disease in patients with chronic renal failure. Nephrol Dial Transplant 9: 1136–1142, 1994.

Canaud B, Béraud JJ, Joyeux H, Mion C. Internal jugular vein cannulation with two silicone rubber catheters: a new and safe temporary vascular access for hemodialysis. 30 months experience. Artif Organs 10: 397–403, 1986.

Canaud B, Bouloux C, Rivory JP, Taib J, Garred LJ, Florence P, Mion C. Erythropoietin-induced changes in protein nutrition: quantitative assessment by urea kinetic modeling analysis. Blood Purif 8: 301–308, 1990.

Chanard J, Bindi P, Lavaud S, Toupance O, Mahent H, Lacour F. Carpal tunnel syndrome and type of dialysis membrane. Br Med J 298: 867–868, 1989.

Charra B, Calemard E, Ruffet M, Chazot C, Terrat JC, Variel T, Laurent G. Survival as an index of adequacy of dialysis. Kidney Int 41: 1286–1291, 1992.

Chatenoud L, Jungers P, Descamps-Latscha B. Immunological considerations of the uremic and dialyzed patient. Kidney Int 45 (suppl 44): S92–S96, 1994.

Chauveau P, Chadefaux B, Coude M, Aupetit J, Hannedouche T, Kamoun P, Jungers P. Hyperhomocysteinemia, a risk factor for atherosclerosis in chronic uremic patients. Kidney Int (suppl 41): S72–S77, 1993.

Cinochowski GE, Worley E, Rutherford WE, Sartain JA, Blondin J, Harter H. Superiority of the internal jugular over the subclavian access for temporary dialysis. Nephron 54: 154–161, 1990.

Combe C, Pourtein M, De Précigout V, et al. Granulocyte activation and adhesion molecules during hemodialysis with cuprophane and a high-flux biocompatible membrane. Am J Kidney Dis 24: 437–442, 1994.

Craddock PR, Fera J, Brigjham KL, Kronenberg PS, Jacob HS. Complement and leucocyte-mediated pulmonary dysfunction in hemodialysis. N Engl J Med 296: 769–774, 1977.

Cressman MD, Heyka RJ, Paganini EP, O'Neil J, Skibinski CI, Hoff HF. Lipoprotein (a) is an independent risk factor for cardiovascular disease in hemodialysis patients. Circulation 86: 475–482, 1992.

Cristol JP, Canaud B, Rabesandratana H, Gaillards I, Serre A, Mion C. Enhancement of reactive oxygen species production and cell surface markers expression due to haemodialysis. Nephrol Dial Transplant 9: 389–394, 1994.

Crosnier J, Jungers P, Couroucé AM, et al. Randomised placebo-controlled trial of hepatitis B surface antigen vaccine in French haemodialysis units. I. Medical Staf; II. Haemodialysis patients. Lancet 1: 455–459 & 797–800, 1981.

Daudon M, Lacour B, Jungers P, et al. Urolithiasis in patients with end stage renal failure. J Urol 147: 977–980, 1992.

Daugirdas JT. Dialysis hypotension: A hemodynamic analysis. Kidney Int 39: 233–246, 1991.

De Broe ME, Druëke TB, Ritz E. Diagnosis and treatment of aluminium overload in end-stage renal failure patients (consensus conference). Nephrol Dial Transplant 8 (suppl 1): 1–54, 1993.
De Marchi S, Cecchin E, Villalta D, Sepiacci G, Santini G, Bartoli E. Relief of pruritus and decreases in plasma histamine concentrations during erythropoietin therapy in patients with uremia. N Engl J Med 326: 969–974, 1992.
Degos F, Jungers P. Dialysis associated hepatitis. In: Jacobs C, Kjellstrand CM, Koch KM, Winchester JF (eds), Replacement of Renal Function by Dialysis, Kluwer Academic Publishers, Dordrecht, The Netherlands, 4th edition, 1995.
Descamps-Latscha B, Herbelin A, Nguyen AT, Zingraff J, Jungers P, Chatenoud L. Immune system dysregulation in uremia. Semin Nephrol 14: 253–260, 1994.
Descamps-Latscha B, Jungers P. Immunological aspects. In: Jacobs C, Kjellstrand CM, Koch KM, Winchester JF (eds), Replacement of Renal Function by Dialysis, Kluwer Academic Publishers, Dordrecht, The Netherlands, 4th edition, 1995.
Dinarello CA. Cytokines: agents provocateurs in hemodialysis? Kidney Int 41: 683–694, 1992.
Dinarello CA. Interleukin-1 and the pathogenesis of the acute-phase reponse. N Engl J Med 311: 1413–1418, 1984.
Drüeke TB, Zingraff J. The dilemma of parathyroidectomy in chronic renal failure. Current Opinion in Nephrology and Hypertension 3: 386–395, 1994.
El-Shahawy MA, Francis R, Akmal M, Massry SG. Recombinant human erythropoietin shortens the bleeding time and corrects the abnormal platelet aggregation in hemodialysis patients. Clin Nephrol 41: 308–313, 1994.
Eschbach JB, Kelley MR, Haley NR, Asys RI, Adamson JW. Treatment of the anemia of progressive renal failure with recombinant human erythropoietin. N Engl J Med 3: 158–163, 1989.
Feest TG, Mistry CD, Grimes DS, Mallick NP. Incidence of advanced chronic renal failure and the need for end stage renal replacement treatment. Br Med J 301: 897–900, 1990.
Fernandez JM, Carbonell ME, Mazzuchi N, Petrucelli D. Simultaneous analysis of morbidity and mortality factors in chronic hemodialysis patients. Kidney Int 41: 1029–1034, 1992.
Foley RN, Parfrey PS, Hefferton D, Singh I, Simms A, Barrett BJ. Advance prediction of early death in patients starting maintenance dialysis. Am J Kidney Dis 23: 836–845, 1994.
Fournier A, Drüeke T, Morinière P, Zingraff J, Boudailliez B, Achard JM. The new treatments of hyperparathyroidism secondary to renal insufficiency. Adv Nephrol 21: 237–306, 1992.
Fournier A, Morinière P, Sebert JL. Calcium carbonate, an aluminium-free agent for control of hyperphosphatemia, hypocalcemia and hyperparathyroidism in uremia. Kidney Int 18: 114–119, 1986.
Fraser CL, Arieff HI. Nervous system complications in uremia. Ann Intern Med 109: 143–153, 1988.
Fujimoto S, Kagoshima T, Hashimoto T, Nakajima T, Dohi K. Left ventricular diastolic function in patients on maintenance hemodialysis: comparison with hypertensive heart disease and hypertrophic cardiomyopathy. Clin Nephrol 42: 109–116, 1994.
Giangrande A, Castiglioni A, Slobiati L, Ballarati E, Caligara F. Chemical

parathyroidectomy for recurrence of secondary hyperparathyroidism. Am J Kidney Dis 24: 421–426, 1994.

Glicklich D. Acquired cystic kidney disease and renal cell carcinoma: A review. Semin Dial 4: 273–283, 1991.

Gomez Campdera FJ, Tejedor A, Orte L. End-stage renal failure therapy in the elderly. Present situation in Spain. Nefrologia 14: 136–144, 1994.

Gotch FA, Sargent JA. A mechanistic analysis of the National Cooperative Dialysis Study (NCDS). Kidney Int 28: 526–534, 1985.

Gutierrez A, Alverstrand A, Wahren J, Bergström J. Effect of in vivo contact between blood and dialysis membranes on protein catabolism in humans. Kidney Int 38: 487–494, 1990.

Haeffner-Cavaillon N, Jacobs G, Poignet JL, Kazatchkine MD. Induction of interleukin-1 during hemodialysis. Kidney Int 43 (suppl 39): S139–S143, 1993.

Hakim RM, Breyer J, Ismail N, Schulman G. Effects of dose of dialysis on morbidity and mortality. Am J Kidney Dis 23: 661–669, 1994.

Hakim RM, Fearon DT, Lazarus JM. Biocompatibility of dialysis membranes: effects of chronic complement activation. Kidney Int 26: 194–200, 1984.

Hakim RM. Assessing the adequacy of dialysis. Kidney Int 37: 822–832, 1990.

Harnett JD, Parfrey PS. Cardiac disease in uremia. Semin Nephrol 14: 245–252, 1994.

Held PJ, Brunner F, Odaka M, Garcia JR, Port FR, Gaylin DS. Five year survival for end-stage renal disease patients in the United States, Europe, and Japan, 1982 to 1987. Am J Kidney Dis 15: 410–413, 1990.

Henderson LW. Solute kinetics and fluid removal in hemofiltration. Int J Artif Organs 6: 5–8, 1983.

Herbelin A, Nguyen AT, Zingraff J, Urena P, Descamps-Latscha B. Influence of uremia and hemodialysis on circulating interleukin-1 and tumor necrosis factor alpha. Kidney Int 37: 116–125, 1990.

Herrmann P, Ritz E, Schmidt-Gayk H, et al. Comparison of intermittent and continuous oral administration of calcitriol in dialysis patients: a randomized prospective trial. Nephron 67: 48–53, 1994.

Hou S, Orlowski J, Pahl M, Ambrose S, Hussey M, Wong D. Pregnancy in women with end-stage renal disease: treatment of anemia and premature labor. Am J Kidney Dis 21: 16–22, 1993.

Hsu CH. The biological action of calcitriol in renal failure. Kidney Int 46: 605–612, 1994.

Iseki K, Kinjo K, Kimura Y, Osawa A, Fukiyama K. Evidence for high risk of cerebral hemorrhage in chronic dialysis patients. Kidney Int 44: 1086–1090, 1993.

Iseki K, Nishime K, Uehara H, Osawa A, Fukiyama K. Effect of renal diseases and comorbid conditions on survival in chronic dialysis patients. Nephron 68: 80–86, 1994.

Jacobs C. Factors limiting optimal dialysis prescription. In: Proc 3rd National Kidney Foundation Clinical Nephrology Meeting, Chicago, April 7–10, pp 82–86, 1994.

Jungers P, Chauveau P, Céballos I, et al. Plasma free aminoacid alterations from early to end-stage chronic renal failure. J Nephrol 7: 48–54, 1994.

Jungers P, Zingraff J, Albouze G, et al. Late referral to maintenance dialysis: detrimental consequences. Nephrol Dial Transplant 8: 1089–1093, 1993.

Jungers P. The progression of renal disease. Kidney, a current survey of world literature 3: 203–208, 1994.

Kaufman JM, Hatzichristou DG, Mulhall JP, Fitch WP, Goldstein I. Impotence and chronic renal failure: a study of the hemodynamic pathophysiology. J Urol 151: 612–618, 1994.

Khan IH, Catto GRD, Edward N, Fleming LW, Henderson IA, Macleod AM. Influence of coexisting disease on survival on renal-replacement therapy. Lancet 341: 415–418, 1993.

Klinkmann H, Davison AM (eds). Consensus conference on biocompatibility. Nephrol Dial Transplant 9 (suppl 2): 1–186, 1994.

Kopple JD, Swendseid E. Protein and amino acid metabolism in uremic patients undergoing maintenance hemodialysis. Kidney Int 7: 64–72, 1975.

Kopple JD. Nutrition, diet and the kidney. In: Shils ME, Young VR (eds), Modern Nutrition in Health and Disease, Malvern, Lea & Febiger, pp 1230–1263, 1988.

Koury MJ. Investigating erythropoietin resistance. N Engl J Med 328: 205–206, 1993.

Lazarus JM, Hakim RM, Newell J. Recombinant human erythropoietin and phlebotomy in the treatment of iron overload in chronic hemodialysis patients. Am J Kidney Dis 16: 101–108, 1990.

Levinsky NG. The organization of medical care. Lessons from the Medicare End Stage Renal Disease program. N Engl J Med 329: 1395–1399, 1993.

Lim VS. Reproductive function in patients with renal insufficiency. Am J Kidney Dis 9: 363–367, 1987.

Lindner A, Charra B, Sherrard DJ, Scribner BH. Accelerated atherosclerosis in prolonged maintenance hemodialysis. N Engl J Med 290: 697–701, 1974.

Lindsay RM, Heidenheim AP, Spanner E, Kortas C, Blake PG. Adequacy of hemodialysis and nutrition: important determinants of morbidity and mortality. Kidney Int 45 (suppl 4): S85–S91, 1994.

London GM, Fabiani F, Marchais SJ, et al. Uremic cardiomyopathy: An inadequate left ventricular hypertrophy. Kidney Int 31: 973–980, 1987.

London GM, Zins B, Pannier BE, et al. Vascular changes in hemodialysis patients in response to recombinant human erythropoietin. Kidney Int 36: 878–882, 1989.

Lowrie EG, Laird NM, Parker TF, Sargent JA. Effect of the hemodialysis prescription on patient morbidity. Report from the National Cooperative Dialysis Study. N Engl J Med 305: 1176–1181, 1981.

Lowrie EG, Lew NL. Death risk in hemodialysis patients: The predictive value of commonly measured variables and an evaluation of death rate differences between facilities. Am J Kidney Dis 15: 458–482, 1990.

Lowrie EG. Chronic dialysis treatment: clinical outcome and related processes of care. Am J Kidney Dis 24: 255–266, 1994.

Mak RHK, De Fronzo RA. Glucose and insulin metabolism in uremia. Nephron 61: 337–342, 1992.

Man NK, Chauveau P, Kuno T, Poignet JL, Yanai M. Phosphate removal during hemodialysis, hemodiafiltration and hemofiltration. Trans Am Soc Artif Intern Organs, 37: M 463–M 465, 1991.

Man NK. Initiation of dialysis: when? Japan J Nephrol 34: 1–8, 1992.

Man NK, Itakura Y, Chauveau P, Yamauchi T. Acetate-free biofiltration: state of the art. In: Maeda K, Shisato T (eds), Effective Hemodiafiltration: New Methods. Contrib Nephrol 108: 87–93, 1994.

Massry SG, Smogorzewski M. Mechanisms through which parathyroid hormone mediates its deleterious effects on organ function in uremia. Semin Nephrol 14: 219–231, 1994.

Massy ZA, Jungers P, Roullet JB, Drüeke T, Lacour B. Disturbances of apolipoprotein distribution in lipoproteins of uremic patients. J. Nephrol 6: 153–158, 1993.

Melhs O, Tonshoff B, Tonshoff C, Haffner D, Blum WF. Therapeutic value of recombinant human growth hormone in children with chronic renal failure. Miner Electrolyte Metab 18: 320–324, 1992.

Mion CM, Hegström RM, Boen ST, Scribner BH. Substitution of sodium acetate for sodium bicarbonate in the bath fluid for hemodialysis. Trans Am Soc Artif Int Organs 10: 107–112, 1964.

Mitch WE, Jurkovitz C, England BK. Mechanisms that cause protein and amino acid catabolism in uremia. Am J Kidney Dis 21: 91–95, 1993.

Movilli E, Mombelloni S, Gaggiotti M, Maiorca R. Effect of age on protein catabolic rate, morbidity, and mortality in uraemic patients with adequate dialysis. Nephrol Dial Transplant 8: 735–739, 1993.

Neu S, Kjellstrand CM. Stopping long-term dialysis: An empirical study of life-supporting treatment. N Engl J Med 314: 14–20, 1986.

Ofsthun NJ, Zydney AL. Importance of convection in artificial kidney treatment. In: Maeda K, Shisato T (eds), Effective Hemodiafiltration: New Methods. Contrib Nephrol 108: 53–70, 1994.

Owen WF, Lew NL, Lin Y, Lowrie EG, Lazarus JM. The urea reduction ratio and serum albumin concentration as predictors of mortality in patients undergoing hemodialysis. N Engl J Med 329: 1001–1006, 1993.

Paganini EP. In search of an optimal hematocrit level in dialysis patients: rehabilitation and quality-of-life implications. Am J Kidney Dis 24 (suppl 1): S10–S16, 1994.

Parfrey PS, Harnett JD. Long-term cardiac morbidity and mortality during dialysis therapy. Adv Nephrol 23: 311–329, 1994.

Parker TF, Husni L, Huang W, Lew N, Lowrie EG, and Dallas Nephrology Associates. Survival of hemodialysis patients in the United States is improved with a greater quantity of dialysis. Am J Kidney Dis 23: 670–680, 1994.

Petitclerc T, Hamani A, Jacobs C. Optimization of sodium balance during hemodialysis by routine implementation of kinetic modeling. Blood Purif 10: 309–316, 1992.

Price R, Mitch WE. Metabolic acidosis and uremic toxicity: Protein and amino acid metabolism. Semin Nephrol 14: 232–237, 1994.

Quarles LD, Lobaugh B, Murphy G. Intact parathyroid hormone overestimates the presence and severity of parathyroid-mediated osseous abnormalities in uremia. J Clin Endocrinol Metab 75: 145–150, 1992.

Quarles LD, Yohay DA, Carroll BA, et al. Prospective trial of pulse oral versus intravenous calcitriol treatment of hyperparathyroidism in ESRD. Kidney Int 45: 1710–1721, 1994.

Quinton W, Dillard D, Scribner BH. Cannulation of blood vessels for prolonged hemodialysis. Trans Am Soc Artif Intern Organs 6: 104–113, 1960.

Raine AEG, Margreiter R, Brunner FP, et al. Report on management of renal failure in Europe, XXII, 1991. Nephrol Dial Transpl 7 (suppl 2): 7–35, 1992.

Raine AEG. Acquired aortic stenosis in dialysis patients. Nephron 68: 159–168, 1994.

Sargent JA, Gotch FA. Mathematical modelling of dialysis therapy. Kidney Int 18 (suppl 10): S2–S10, 1980.
Shaldon S, Beau MC, Deschodt G, Ramperez P, Mion C. Vascular stability during hemofiltration. Trans Am Soc Artif Intern Organs 26: 391–393, 1980.
Shaldon S. Reuse of haemodialysers. Nephrol Dial Transplant 9: 1226–1227, 1994.
Sherrard D, Hercz G, Pei Y, et al. The spectrum of bone disease in end-stage renal failure – An evolving disorder. Kidney Int 43: 436–442, 1993.
Silbelberg JS, Barre PE, Prichard SS, et al. Impact of left ventricular hypertrophy on survival in end stage renal disease. Kidney Int 36: 286–290, 1989.
Slatopolsky E, Weerts C, Norwood K, et al. Long-term effects of calcium carbonate and 2.5 mEq/liter calcium dialysate on mineral metabolism. Kidney Int 36: 897–903, 1989.
Sprenger KB, Kratz W, Lewis AE, Stadtmuller U. Kinetic modeling of hemodialysis, hemofiltration and hemodiafiltration. Kidney Int 24: 143–151, 1983.
Stewart CL, Fine RN. Growth in children with renal insufficiency. Semin Dial 6: 37–45, 1993.
Terasawa Y, Suzuki Y, Morita M, Kato M, Suzuki K, Sekino H. Ultrasonic diagnosis of renal cell carcinoma in hemodialysis patients. J Urol 152: 846–851, 1994.
United States Renal Data System. The 1993 USRDS annual data report. Am J Kidney Dis 22 (suppl 4): 1–115, 1993.
Urena P, Herbelin A, Zingraff J, Man NK, Descamps-Latscha B, Drüeke T. Permeability of cellulosic and non-cellulosic membranes to endotoxin subunits and cytokine production during in-vitro haemodialysis. Nephrol Dial Transplant 7: 16–28, 1992.
Valderrabano F, on behalf of the EDTA Registry. Figures from annual report on management of renal failure in Europe, XXIV, 1993. Proc XXXIth Congress of EDTA-ERA, Vienna, 3–6 July 1994.
Valderrabano F. Nutrition and quality of hemodialysis. Nefrologia 14 (suppl 2): 2–13, 1994.
Van Ypersele de Strihou C, Jadoul M, Malghem J, et al. Effect of dialysis membrane and patient's age on signs of dialysis-related amyloidosis. Kidney Int 39: 1012–1019, 1991.
Vanholder R, De Smet R, Hsu C, Vogeleere P, Ringoir S. Uremic toxicity: The middle molecule hypothesis revisited. Semin Nephrol 14: 205–218, 1994.
Vanholder R, Ringoir S. Adequacy of dialysis: A critical review. Kidney Int 42: 540–558, 1992.
Vanholder R, Ringoir S. Infectious morbidity and defects of phagocytic function in end-stage renal disease: a review. J Am Soc Nephrol 3: 1541–1554, 1993.
Vaziri ND, Gonzales EC, Wang J, Said S. Blood coagulation, fibrinolytic and inhibitory proteins in end-stage renal disease: effect of hemodialysis. Am J Kidney Dis 23: 828–835, 1994.
Williams B, Walls J. Metabolic acidosis: a significant catabolic factor in chronic renal failure. J Nephrol 7: 73–76, 1994.
Williams ME. Insulin management of a diabetic patient on hemodialysis. Semin Dial 5: 69–73, 1992.
Zaoui PM, Stone WJ, Hakim RM. Effects of dialysis membranes on $\beta 2$-microglobulin production and cellular expression. Kidney Int 38: 962–968, 1990.

Zingraff J, Jungers P, Pelissier C, Nahoul K, Feinstein MC, Scholler R. Pituitary and ovarian dysfunction in women on haemodialysis. Nephron 30: 149–153, 1982.

Zingraff J, Drüeke T. Can the nephrologist prevent dialysis-related amyloidosis? Am J Kidney Dis, 18: 1–11, 1991.

SUBJECT INDEX

Accelerated atherosclerosis **73–74**
ACE inhibitors (ACEI) 45, 46, 70
Acetate buffer 37
Acetate-associated side-effects 37, 66, 67
Acetate-free biofiltration 16
Acetate-induced hypoxemia 67
Acidosis 100
Acquired cystic disease of the kidneys 103
Acrylonitrile copolymers 32
Activated charcoal filter 39
Activation of blood components 42
Adequacy of dialysis **49–60**
Adequate dialysis criteria 49
Adsorption 13
Adynamic bone disease 94
Age of ESRD patients 3, 110
Air detector 35
Air embolism 65
Albumin, serum level of 52, 54
Alfacalcidol 92
Alkaline phosphatase 91
Allogenous veins (for AV fistula) 24
Allopurinol 97
Aluminum encephalopathy 77
Aluminum-containing phosphate binders 91, 93
Aluminum-related osteomalacia 93, 94
Aluminum toxicity **93–94**
Amenorrhea 99
Aminoacid losses in dialysis 39
Amyloid cysts 95
AN69 membranes 32

Anaphylactoid reactions 45
Anaphylatoxins 45
Anemia **84–87**
Aneurysmal development of AV fistula 27
Angina pectoris 66, 72, 74
Angiodysplasia 102
Angiography of AV fistula 25
Angiotensin converting enzyme (ACE) 46
Angiotensin converting enzyme inhibitors 45,46
Anorexia 5, 55
Anticardiolipin antibodies 26
Anticoagulation 31
Antihypertensive therapy 70
Anxiety 104
Aortic stenosis 75
Aplastic bone disease 88, 94
Apolipoproteins 100
Arrhythmia during dialysis 66
Arteriovenous fistula 22
Arteriovenous grafts 23
Arteritis 73
Atherosclerosis **73–74**
Autogenous vein grafts 23

Backfiltration 19
Bacterial infections 26, 81
Bacterial lipopolysaccharides 42
Basic principles of dialysis **11–21**
Beta 2-microglobulin 47, 95
Beta 2-microglobulin amyloidosis **94–96**

Bicarbonate-buffered dialysis 37, 67
Biocompatibility **42–48**
Biocompatible membranes 44
Biofilm 36
Biofiltration 16
Bleeding disorders 87
Blood access **22–28**
Blood-born viral infections 84
Blood compartment resistance 12
Blood flow rate (in AV fistula) 23, 27
Blood flow rate (in dialyzer) 16
Blood leak detector 35
Blood losses 31, 84
Blood restitution 64
Blood urea nitrogen (BUN) 5
Bone biopsy 88, 91, 93
Bovine carotid artery 24
Bradykinin 45
Bullous dermatoses 101

Calcifediol 92
Calcitriol 7, 89, 92
Calcium acetate 92
Calcium carbonate 92
Calcium citrate 77,93
Calcium concentration in dialysate 36, 92
Calcium-containing phosphate binders 91, 92
Calcium set-point 89
Calorie-protein requirement 57
Carbohydrate metabolism disorders 100
Carbon filters 40
Carboxymethylpropylfuranpropionic acid 6
Cardiac arrhythmias 66
Cardiac dysfunction **71–72**
Cardiomyopathy 71
Cardiovascular problems **69–76**
Carpal tunnel syndrome 95
Causes of ESRD **1–4**
Cellulose acetate 32
Cellulose diacetate 32
Cellulose triacetate 32
Cellulosic membranes 31
Center hemodialysis 67

Central vein catheters 27
Cerebral hemorrhage 77
Cerebrovascular accidents 77
Chemical structure of membranes 31
Chest pain 66
Children (dialysis in) **104–105**
Chloramines 6, 40
Chloride concentration in dialysate 38
Chronic glomerulonephritis 2
Cimino-Brescia fistula 22
Citrate ion, and aluminium absorption 77, 93
Clearance of dialyzers 16
Clinical surveillance of dialysis session 64
Clotting of blood access 25, 27
Coagulation in the blood circuit 31
Cockcroft-Gault formula 8
Comorbidity (comorbid conditions) 2, 108
Complement activating membranes 42
Complement activation **42–44**
Complications of blood access **25–27**
Computerized monitoring 35
Concentration gradient 12
Conductimetry 35
Conduction (or diffusion) 11
Congestive heart failure 72
Conjugated estrogens 87
Constipation 102
Convection 12
Convective transfer 12, 19
Convulsions 61, 65
Coronarography 73, 74
Coronary artery disease **73–74**
Cost of dialysis therapy **111–112**
Cramps 66
Creatinine 5
Creatinine clearance 8
Criteria for initiating dialysis 8
Criteria of adequate dialysis 49
Cryoprecipitate 87
Cuprophan membranes 31, 44
Cystic kidney disease (acquired) 91
Cytokines 45, 80

Declotting of vascular access 25
Deferoxamine chelation therapy 94
Deferoxamine test 93
Depression 104
Dermatological problems 100
Desmopressin 87
Diabetic nephropathy 2,3
Diabetic patients (dialysis in) **106–107**
Dialysance (of dialyzers) 17
Dialysate composition **36–39**
Dialysate delivery systems **33–36**
Dialysis dementia 77
Dialysis disequilibrium syndrome 61
Dialysis dose 50
Dialysis duration **54–57**
Dialysis equipment **29–41**
Dialysis membranes **31–32**
Dialysis prescription **56–57**
Dialyzers **29–31**
Dialyzer performances 16
Diastolic dysfunction 71
Dietary prescription **57–59**
Dietary record 58
Diffusion (or conduction) 11
Digitalis 66, 72
Dilated cardiomyopathy 71
Dimethylarginine 6
Disinfection procedures **36**
Distal ischemia 27
Diverticulitis 81, 102
Doppler velocimetry of AV fistula 25
Double-lumen catheters 27
Drug-protein binding 6
Dry weight 63, 65, 70
Dysgueusia 102
Dyslipidemia 100

Early placement of vascular access 9, 28
Echocardiography 71
Economic issues **110–112**
Elderly patients (dialysis in) **106**
Encephalopathy 76
End-stage renal disease (ESRD) 1
Endocarditis 75
Endocrine disorders **99**

Endocrine functions of the kidneys 7
Endotoxins 40, 46
Epidemiology of chronic renal failure **1–4**
Equipment for hemodialysis **29–41**
Erectile dysfunction 99
Erythropoietin 7, 84
Ethylene oxide (ETO) 45
Ethylvinyl alcohol (EVAL) 32
Excessive flow rate of blood access 27
Excretory functions of the kidneys **5–7**

Femoral vein catheterization 27
Ferritin 85
Fever (prolonged) 82
Fibrous osteitis **88–90**
First hemodialysis session 59
First-use syndrome 46
Fistulography 25
Flat-plate dialyzers 29
Flow rate in AV fistula 23
Flow rate of blood 56
Flow rate of dialysate 56
Fluid intake of the dialysis patient 58
Fluid overload 67
Fluid removal 63
Fluorosis 98
Folic acid supplementation 59
Fructosamine 107

Gastro-intestinal bleeding 102
Gastroduodenal ulcer 102
Gastro-intestinal complications **102–103**
General continuous heparinization 62
General discontinuous heparinization 62
General precautions against viral infections 84
Glomerular filtration rate (GFR) 1
Glomerulonephritis 2
Glucose concentration in dialysate 38
Glucose intolerance 100

Glycosylated hemoglobin 95
Gout 6, 97
Gram-negative infections 81
Granulomatosis 103
Growth hormone 105
Guanidine compounds 6
Guanidinosuccinic acid 6

Hageman factor 45
Hard-water syndrome 65
Headache 61
Heart failure 72
Hemasite device 25
Hematological problems **84–87**
Hematuria 103
Hemodiafiltration 15
Hemodialysis-related hypotension **65–67**
Hemodialytic solute transport 14
Hemodynamic instability **65–66**, 74
Hemofiltration 14
Hemolysis (acute) 66
Hemophan 31
Hemosiderosis 86
Heparinization 62
Hepatitis **83–84**
Hepatitis B vaccine 83
Hepatitis B virus 83
Hepatitis C virus 83, 84
High-flux dialyzers 30
High-flux membranes 32
High-output cardiac failure 23, 27
High-permeability membranes 30
High-turnover bone disease 88, 91
Hippuric acid 6
Hollow-fiber dialyzers 29
Home dialysis 67
Homocysteine 6, 100
Hormonal functions of the kidney **7**
Human immunodeficiency virus (HIV) 84
Hydraulic permeability 13, 18, 32
Hydroelectrolytic regulation 7
Hydrophilic membranes 32
Hydrophobic membranes 13, 32
Hydrosoluble vitamins 59
Hydrostatic pressure 18, 19
Hydroxyl groups 42
Hypercalcemia 92

Hypercoagulability 25
Hyperhomocysteinemia 59, 73, 100
Hyperkalemia 67
Hypernatremia 65
Hyperparathyroidism **89–92**
Hyperphosphatemia 89, 92
Hyperprolactinemia 99
Hypertension **70–71**
Hypertensive nephrosclerosis 2
Hyperthermia 65
Hypertonic dialysate 65
Hypertriglyceridemia 100
Hypoalbuminemia 53
Hypocalcemia 89
Hypochromic anemia 85
Hyponatremia 65
Hyporesponsiveness to r-HuEPO 86
Hypotension in hemodialysis sessions **65–67**
Hypotonic dialysate 65
Hypoxemia during hemodialysis 67

IgA nephropathy 1
Immune system dysregulation **78–80**
Immunoactivation 78, 79
Immunodeficiency 69
Impotence 99
Incidence of ESRD **2–3**
Incidents during dialysis sessions **64–67**
Increasing needs for dialysis therapy 110
Indications for initiating dialysis **7–10**
Indoles 6
Indoxyl sulfate 6
Infection of vascular access 26
Infectious problems **81–84**
Infertility 99
Inflammatory disorders 47, 48
Initiation of dialysis therapy 8
Insulin resistance 100
Integrated dialysis prescription **59–60**
Interdialytic complications **67**
Interdialytic weight gain 58, 63
Interleukin 1 (IL-1) 43, 45, 80
Interleukin 2 (IL-2) 79, 80

Internal jugular vein catheter 27
Interstitial nephritis **2**
Intradialytic hazards **64–67**
Ionized calcium 79
Iron deficiency 85, 86
Iron overload 82, 86, 101
Iron supplementation 85
Ischemic colitis 102
Ischemic heart disease 71

Kallikrein cascade 45
Kidney diseases leading to ESRF **1–2**
Kidney stones 104
Kt/V (definition) **49**
Kt/V urea 50, 54

Laboratory surveillance of the dialysis patient 68
Large surface-area dialyzers 30
Left ventricular dysfunction 71
Left ventricular hypertrophy 71
Length of survival in dialysis **108**
Leukopenia during dialysis 44
Libido 99
Limited-care hemodialysis 68
Lipid metabolism disorders 100
Lipopolysaccharides (LPS) 42
Listeria monocytogenes 82
Liver biopsy 84
Low-turnover bone disease 88, 93
Low calcium dialysate 92
Low molecular weight heparin 62
Low-molecular weight toxins 5
Luteal insufficiency 99

Macrocytic anemia 85
Magnesium concentration in dialysate 38
Malnutrition 53
Management of the dialysis patient **61–68**
Mass solute transfer **2**
Meals during hemodialysis 63
Membranes **31–32**
Menorrhagia 99
Metabolic disorders **100**
Metastatic calcifications 96
Methylguanidine 6

Microbial contamination 42
Microcrystalline arthropathy 97
Microcytic anemia 93
Middle molecular weight toxins 6
Monitoring devices 35
Monitoring of blood circuit 35
Monitoring of dialysate 35
Monitoring of ultrafiltration 35
Monocyte activation 80
Morbidity in dialysis **51–53**
Mortality in dialysis **51–53**
Mucormycosis 94
Muscle cramps 66, 76
Myocardial infarction 69, 73
Myoinisitol 6

National Cooperative Dialysis Study (NCDS) 51
Nausea 5, 66
Nausea during dialysis 66
Needle puncture 62
Negatively charged membranes 45, 70
Nerve conduction velocity 76
Neurologic problems **76–77**
Neuropathy 76
Neutropenia 44,
Neutrophil sequestration 44
Nitrates 40
Nitric oxide 70
Non complement activating membranes 44
Non substituted cellulose membranes 31, 45, 67
Non urea nitrogen (NUN) 52, 53
Nosocomial transmission 83
Nutritional parameters and outcome 53
Nutritional parameters of dialysis adequacy 52
Nutritional prescription **58–59**
Nutritional status 52

Obstructive nephropathy 2
Omeprazole 102
Opportunistic infections 81
Optimal dialysis conditions 110
Optimal dialysis duration **56**

Osmotic pressure 13
Osteitis fibrosa **88–90**
Osteoarticular problems **88–98**
Osteodystrophy (renal) **88–96**
Osteomalacia 93
Osteoporosis 97
Overheated dialysate 65, 66
Oxalate 6
Oxidants 80

Paired-filtration dialysis 16
Pancreatitis 103
Parallel-plate dialyzers 29, 30
Parathyroidectomy 92
Parathyroid hormone (PTH) 89
Pediatric dialysis **104–105**
Peptic ulcer 102
Percutaneous transluminal angioplasty 25
Performances of dialyzers **16–19**
Pericarditis 74, 75
Permeability characteristics of membranes 32
Phagocytic activity 79
Phosphate retention 89
Phosphate binders 91
Pituitary-gonadal axis 99
Platelet dysfunction 87
Polyacrylonitrile (PAN) 32
Polyamide (PA) 32, 44
Polyamines 6
Polycarbonate (PC) 32
Polycystic kidney disease 81
Polymethylmethacrylate (PMMA) 32
Polymorphonuclear neutrophils 79
Polysufone (PS) 32
Polytetrafluoroethylene (PTFE) 24
Polyunsaturated fats 100
Porphyria cutanea tarda 101
Porphyrins 101
Postdilution mode (hemofiltration) 15
Potassium in dialysate 36
Prealbumin 52
Predilution mode (hemofiltration) 13
Pregnancy in ESRD patients 99
Preparation to dialysis 8

Pressure gradient 10,13
Professional activity 110
Progression of renal failure 9
Proinflammatory cytokines 45, 80
Prolonged fever 82
Proteases 80
Protein C 26
Protein catabolic rate (PCR) 52, 53
Protein catabolism 41
Protein intake 53, 56
Protein requirement 57
Protein S 26
Protoporphyrins 101
Pruritus 100
Pseudoporphyria 101
Psychological preparation 9
Psychological problems 104
Pulmonary edema 67
Pulmonary leukocyte sequestration 67
Purines 6
Push-pull hemofiltration 14
Pyridoxin 59
Pyrogens 40

Quality of life (QOL) **109–110**
Quinton-Scribner shunt 22

Radiocephalic AV fistula 22
Reactive oxygen species (ROS) 43, 45, 80
Recirculation 25
Recombinant human erythropoietin (r-HuEPO) **85–86**
Recombinant human growth hormone (r-HuGH) 105
Recommended target Kt/V value 56
Refilling rate 65
Reflux nephropathy 2
Regenerated cellulose 31
Rehabilitation **109–110**
Renal cell carcinoma, acquired 103
Renal osteodystrophy **88–96**
Renal transplantation 10, 111
Renin-angiotensin axis 7
Renin-dependent hypertension 70
Repeated clotting of vascular access 25
Residual blood volume 31

Residual diuresis 7, 57
Resistance to erythropoietin therapy 86
Resistance to solute transfer 12
Restless legs syndrome 76
Reuse of dialyzers 31
Reverse osmosis 40, 41

Saphenous vein allografts 23
Saphenous vein autografts 23
Scribner's shunt 22
Selenium deficiency 69
Self-care hemodialysis 68
Semipermeable membranes 11
Serum albumin **53–54**
Set-point of calcium 89
Sieving coefficient **12–14**, 20
Single-needle dialysis 62
Single-pass dialysate 17
Sodium concentration in dialysate 36
Sodium intake 58
Sodium modeling 35
Softeners 39, 41
Soft tissue calcifications 96, 97
Solute mass removal **20–21**
Solute transport **11–16**
Splanchnic vasodilation 64
Spondylarthropathy 98
Squeletal resistance to parathormone 89
Staphylococcal infections 81
Staphylococcus aureus 26, 81
Staphylococcus epidermidis 26, 81
Steal syndrome 27
Stenosis of AV fistula 25
Stent in AV fistula 26
Sterile dialysate 48
Subclavian vein catheter 27
Subdural hematoma 77
Subtotal parathyroidectomy 82
Substitution fluid for hemofiltration 15
Surveillance of dialysis sessions **64**
Survival rate on hemodialysis **109**
Systemic diseases 2
Systolic dysfunction 71

Tamponade (cardiac) 75

Technical hazards during hemodialysis sessions **64–67**
Telangiectasias 102
Temporary vascular access **27–28**
Termination of treatment 92
Thomas shunt 25
Thrombogenicity of dialyzers 31
Thrombolysis 25
Thyroid hormones 99
Time-averaged urea concentration (TAC) 51
Total body water 50
Transfer of solutes **11–16**
Transfusion 86
Transmembrane pressure 13, 16
Transplantation 2
Transport mechanisms **11–16**
Transposition (of veins) 23
Tuberculosis 82
Tumor necrosis factor (TNFα) 43
Tunnelized catheters 27

Ultrafiltration 18
Ultrafiltration control devices 30
Underdialysis 53
Unsaturated fats 100
Unsubstituted cellulosic membranes 31, 47
Urea 5
Urea extraction and clinical outcome 51
Urea kinetic modeling 49
Urea monitors 21
Urea reduction ratio (URR) 50, 53
Uremia **1**
Uremic encephalopathy 76
Uremic polyneuropathy 76
Uremic syndrome **4–7**
Uric acid 5

Vaccination against HBV 83
Vaccination responses 79
Valvular heart disease 75
Vascular connexion 62
Vascular steal syndrome 27
Vicious circle from underdialysis to undernutrition 55
Viral hepatitis **82–84**
Virus B hepatitis 83

Virus C hepatitis 83, 84
Vitamin B12 (clearance) 18
Vitamin D 89, 92
Vitamin supplements 59
Volume control 63
Volume-dependent hypertension 70
Vomiting 5, 66

Warm dialysate 65, 66

Water treatment **39–41**
Weekly dialysis time 56, 110
Weight loss during dialysis sessions 63
Withdrawal of dialysis therapy 104

Yersinia enterolytica 82, 94

Zinc deficiency 78